Autism - The Road to Recovery
(Dr. Kurt N. Woeller's Autism Action Plan)

An Autism Recovery Guide
for Parents and Physicians

By
Kurt N. Woeller, D.O.

www.AutismActionPlan.com
www.DrWoeller.com

Table of Contents

The Regressive Autism Child

- Comprehensive Biomedical Approach to Testing & Treatment

- The Roots of Biomedical Therapy for Autism
- Basic Overview of Biomedicine for Autism
- The Biomedical Approach – Incorporates Many Aspects of Medicine

- Do you Believe Your Child's Autism-Spectrum Disorder Stems From a Toxicity Issue (aka. Medical Problem) and is Not Just a Developmental Brain Disorder?
- Asking the Question
- Yes or No! What Do You Do Now?
- Bottom Line – Again

- Getting Informed and Maintaining an Open Mind
- Understanding the 4 Major Categories of Treatment

- Low Oxalate Diet
- Feingold Program, Phenol and Salicylate Sensitivity
- So Where to Begin

- What is Methylation
- Genetics of Methylation Problems in Autistic Individuals
- Methylcobalamin (MB-12) Therapy – The Gold Standard Approach
- What Are the Benefits You Can Expect from Methyl-B12 Injections?
- Any Physician Can Order Methyl-B12
- Methyl-B12 Dosing Specifics and Instructions
- Other Recommendations
- What Are the Common Side Effects from Methyl-B12 Injections?
- Other Forms of Methyl-B12

- Scientific Rationale Behind Respen-A™

Additional Information:

Preface

I am often asked how I began working with children with autism-spectrum disorders. My response is always the same. The autism community found me, I did not find them.

In 1998, while working at a health clinic in San Diego, CA, I received an advertisement in the mail for something called a DAN! (Defeat Autism Now!) conference (now called the Autism Research Institute Conferences). My office partner mentioned we should go see what the presenting doctors had to say about this condition called Autism. Not having any formal understanding of autism (other than the movie "Rain Man"), I went, anticipating learning something new. I was not disappointed. Listening to the various lectures, I realized that the Autism-spectrum health conditions these doctors were talking about were many of the same things I was seeing in my general patient population, such as mental/emotional disorders, lack of focus and concentration, digestive problems, immune dysfunction, food sensitivities, nutritional imbalances and deficiencies. I was intrigued, and a bit overwhelmed by the information, but was willing to help children if they found their way to my office. I soon realized that would not take very long.

The following weeks after the conference, I started getting phone calls asking if I was treating autism. My response to the office staff was one of bewilderment. How were these people finding me? I had not advertised nor even spoken to anyone about my attendance at the autism conference. As it turned out, when I registered for the conference, I had filled out a form asking if I would be willing to be a DAN! practitioner. I must have marked "yes", and from that point on, my name was added to the Autism Research Institutes practitioner referral list. Things happened quickly as I was suddenly thrust into the world of biomedical assessment and treatment of autism-spectrum individuals (children, teenagers and adults). Since my first patient with autism, the journey has been one of intense study, challenges, dedication, and exploration. I have seen many wonderful changes happen with people on the road to recovery, and have had the opportunity to work with many dedicated parents trying to help their loved ones with autism.

My work has also brought frustration and anger at a medical system that has allowed this condition to reach epidemic proportions. We are truly in the midst of a catastrophic crisis with regards to neuro-development disorders, not only here in the United States, but worldwide.

Unfortunately, the situation is getting worse, but as doctors dedicated to biomedical intervention for autism, we have many more tools at our disposal, such as nutritional support, dietary interventions, heavy metal detoxification therapies, immune enhancing products including medications, herbal and homeopathic remedies and more. I believe *all* individuals, including adults and children dealing with this disorder can benefit by biomedical approaches to their health condition.

I feel blessed to have the opportunity to help people in need. There is much that can be done. The road to recovery is not always easy. Many sacrifices must be made with regards to lifestyle changes, diet, therapeutic interventions, time, and resources. However, the end result of improved health for those with autism is well worth the effort. As a physician, I see myself as a facilitator and educator in this process. I also feel it's my duty to expand my knowledge and have the willingness to explore new avenues of treatment.

Finally, as a father of two children, I see the potential in their eyes for a bright and happy future. As a physician, father, and fellow human being, I feel honored to work with dedicated parents in a mutual goal to bring their loved one back from the darkness of autism. This goal is achievable and my mission is to never give up in making it reality for people suffering with this devastating condition. What others have said is impossible, is achievable, if you stay the course and believe that people suffering with autism can get better. I truly believe they can.

Sincerely,
Kurt N. Woeller, D.O.

3

Introduction

The purpose for this book is to address what I feel are the important issues you, as a parent or caregiver, need to know about in implementing a biomedical approach for your loved one (child, teenager or adult) with an autism-spectrum disorder.

My biomedical approach incorporates many different facets of medicine, including diagnostic testing, dietary and lifestyle modifications, nutritional, herbal and homeopathic supplements. In addition, certain medications (if needed), such as antiviral, antibacterial, anti-parasitic therapy, anti-fungals like Nystatin or Diflucan, Respen-A, Namenda, and others, plus traditional heavy metal detoxifiers such as EDTA, DMPS, DMSA, as well as specialized therapies like methylcobalamin (Methyl-B12), folinic acid and methyl-folate, and hyperbaric oxygen therapy, may be necessary. My understanding is that the majority of autism-spectrum individuals, including those with attention deficit (ADD) and attention deficit hyperactivity disorder (ADHD) and other neurodevelopment problems are dealing with underlying biological and toxicity issues (i.e. chemical, heavy metal, food, infections) that are compromising their health. Autism and its related spectrum disorders are more than just a psychological (or neurodevelopment disorder) condition without hope for recovery or improvement. In fact, physicians using the biomedical approach feel that the majority of people who are treated have a significant chance of improvement, if not full recovery (particularly children).

My approach with autism stems from a biomedical viewpoint. I feel the best chance a person has at "optimizing their full potential" is to incorporate biomedical therapies along with standard therapies such as behavioral, speech, auditory processing, and occupational therapy.

The biomedical approach is too important to leave out of any treatment program no matter how old they are, or how long they have been diagnosed with autism. Even those who do not have an official diagnosis, but clearly have an issue the same or similar to others on the spectrum can derive benefit. Health can always be improved and my goal is to optimize an individual's potential with the ultimate goal of a possible complete recovery. However, implementing biomedical therapies takes work and dedication on your part as a parent or caregiver. There are no "quick fixes," nor magic bullets. Consistent and simultaneous implementation of a variety of biomedical therapies is needed for optimal success.

The most important task for you as a parent or caregiver is to become knowledgeable about the variety of biomedical therapies available. My focus in this book is to provide you with useful information to help you get started in this process. The amount of information related to the biomedical approach can be overwhelming, and the list of available therapeutics keeps growing. Knowing what to do first, how to prioritize testing, therapies, dietary changes, and which supplements to use leaves many parents feeling overwhelmed and frustrated. This is understandable because much of the information that is available about biomedical intervention is not well recognized by the traditional medical community. Much of the information needs to be obtained from books, articles, websites, support groups and other internet resources.

This lack of information through conventional medical channels does not mean the biomedical approach has no value. In fact, it is absolutely essential, but don't expect to get much recognition or support from closed minded physicians or other health care providers. They have ignored the problem for years and do not offer much hope for effective treatment or improvement for your loved one. Instead, focus on the potential that biomedical therapy has to offer.

Explore the avenue of hope that many parents have discovered as they watch their children undergo significant improvement and even recovery from their autism-spectrum diagnosis.

Traditional medicine has no 100% guarantees for absolute recovery from any illness - neither does a biomedical approach to autism make any such guarantees. However, my goal is to help each person reach their full health potential whatever their potential is destined to be.

My approach is taken in steps or phases of assessment and treatment. The initial phase begins with diagnostic testing which is covered extensively in Chapter 7. Assessment is always necessary first in order to start more specific therapies such as metal detoxification or anti-yeast treatment. However, there are many things that you can do initially to begin helping your loved one. This involves the process of self-education and the understanding of how biomedical treatment programs work. Education is power! The more you read and expose yourself to new ways of thinking the better able you will be in making informed decisions regarding treatment. Chapter 6 gives some detailed information about articles, support groups, conferences/seminars and other books that I recommend for deepening your knowledge base.

Chapter 9 explores one of the most beneficial therapies in my experience called Methyl-B12 therapy; while Chapter 5 discusses how to implement the various Action Steps.

There is also a chapter on Respen-A (Chapter 10). This therapy (available since 2008) is extremely helpful and effective in my experience. More information is available online from my subscription website at www.AutismActionPlan.com through the Parent Forum. This website provides access to me personally for day-to-day questions and answers regarding biomedical intervention for autism.

I hope you find this book informative and use it as a resource for helping your loved one with autism. My action plan has been developed over time from working with patients, many of them with complex health issues. My action plan has been influenced by the Defeat Autism Now! (DAN!) organization, including the Autism Research Institute and the late Dr. Bernard Rimland, and its wonderful group of health professionals, as well as other influential physicians and health providers dedicated to treating children and adults with autism including Bill Timmins, N.D., Jim Jealous, D.O., James Neubrander, M.D., William Shaw, Ph. D. and many, many more.

Also, I cannot forget the parents. It is the parents who are the driving force behind the implementation of biomedical therapies. Some of the greatest teachers I have are parents themselves working tirelessly to improve the life of their

loved one with autism. I wish you knowledge, health, success, and happiness in this journey to recovery for your loved one from the clutches of autism.
Kurt N. Woeller, D.O.
www.AutismActionPlan.com
www.DrWoeller.com

About the Use of the Term "Autism" in This Book

My use of the word "autism" throughout this book is meant to encompass all individuals with an autism-spectrum diagnosis. It is not to convey that those with an official diagnosis can only be helped. There are many individuals with spectrum problems who do not have an official autism diagnosis, but can still be greatly helped by the information in the book.

Also, I will refer to autism, as "autism kids, children or children with autism or an autism-spectrum disorder" to be all inclusive for older individuals as well, including teenagers and adults. Please realize that the majority of individuals with an autism-spectrum disorder can be helped with biomedical intervention – not just children.

Finally, I will often throughout this book refer to autism as autism, autism-spectrum, autism-spectrum disorder or simply ASD.

Chapter 1
A Typical Child Diagnosed with Autism

"My husband George and I were ecstatic with the birth of our first child, Robert. He was a lively, happy and an adorable child. He was also healthy, thriving and appeared absolutely normal. Then suddenly...at about 18 months...he went away..."

I have interviewed hundreds and hundreds of families who tell a similar story to that listed above. They come from all nationalities, environments and socioeconomic backgrounds. However, none of this seems to matter. What is common to many children with autism is the way in which autism seemingly overtook them. Often there is a pattern to their autism - events that likely contributed to their eventual diagnosis. I am going to describe to you the common pattern of *regressive* autism that I have seen in my practice. However, don't think that if your child does not fall into this category that they cannot be helped by biomedical therapies - <u>any</u> and <u>every</u> child (including teenagers and adults) can be helped with biomedical intervention.

NOTE: I will use "he" or "his" and "child" for either gender.

The Regressive Autism Child

This pattern of development is only an example, but many of the issues listed below are common to most regressive cases of autism that I have seen.

- The child is born seemingly healthy, either via C-section or vaginal delivery. Pitocin is often used to assist with labor.
- No apparent issues at birth – he may or may not have received hepatitis B vaccine.
- At age two months the child received his first series of vaccines.
- Within the first three to four months the child is diagnosed with an ear infection. Oral antibiotics are prescribed.
- The child may successfully breast feed for three to four months, then is switched to formula – usually soy based.
- A second ear infection is diagnosed at around four to five months – again another round of oral antibiotics.
- He begins eating solids at about six months. More antibiotics are given for an unresolved ear infection.
- Then come the four and six month vaccines. However, he continues to develop normally. He's playful, appears happy and content, and eye contact appears intact.
- Possibly another course of antibiotics is given prior to the first birthday because of continuous ear infections.
- At one year the child is switched from breast milk or formula to cow dairy.

- He continues good progress developmentally, including verbalizing the words "dada" and/or "mama."
- Ear infections and allergies become more prominent. More antibiotics are given.
- The child begins to have loose stools after cow dairy is implemented.
- Between the 12th and 15th month of age he receives another round of vaccines, including the MMR and chicken pox vaccines.
- Parents begin to notice a marked change in stool patterns, including an increase of diarrhea, light colored stools and "sandy-like" substance in his stools.
- Between 15 to 18 months he begins to lose words, no-longer saying "dada" or "mama." He appears to be deaf as he no longer responds to his name.
- The child starts to fixate on spinning objects, i.e. fans, the wheels on toy cars or trucks.
- This pattern usually takes about two to three months to develop, but in some cases it happens over hours, days or a few weeks.
- By the time the child is 18 to 20 months old he is no longer communicative. He appears isolated and withdrawn. Diarrhea continues.
- More ear infections keep emerging despite repeated courses of antibiotics.
- The parents are told by their pediatrician that most kids go through a transition period in their toddler years, and that boys will many times have delays in language.
- This cycle continues until it is evident that the child is not developing normally, but instead is losing ground compared to other children their age with respect to speech, socialization, etc.

- The child is eventually diagnosed with an autism-spectrum disorder and provided various services to help with education, speech and behavioral therapies.
- No significant medical therapies are investigated or implemented, except for basic genetic screening for Fragile X or cursory blood work. Often times this doesn't even happen. Most of the time these tests are normal.
- Parents concerns regarding the child's health, diarrhea, potential vaccine reactions, etc. are disregarded.

I realize this is a simplistic outline of a child's regression into autism. Some children regress much more quickly even before their first birthday. Some never develop language or only partially lose it. Some parents describe their child as never developing normally, or always appearing delayed. There are a variety of scenarios, but with respect to the regressive pattern (which makes up approximately 70 to 80 percent of the kids in my practice) the general pattern is the same – normal development, seemingly appropriate socialization skills for their age, language development on target and then suddenly something happens. What was gained is lost. What never developed is never seen. The typical child regresses into a world of isolation.

I have seen this pattern over and over for years now. Many biomedical autism doctors can predict, based on a brief history of the child, what are likely the contributing factors to the child's underlying health issues. As an example, I have seen kids regress into autism days after a series of vaccines – one in particular is the combined Measles, Mumps, and

Rubella (MMR), which in my opinion is a significant culprit in regressive autism (regardless of what the media states…they are flat out wrong in my opinion) – it is not the only culprit, but a significant one.

Approaching Autism as a Medical Issue

As a parent or caregiver you obviously have your own story to tell about your child. Their particular pattern may have been entirely different from what I have listed above, or incorporated some of what was listed. What is important is that you are beginning to look at what may have been contributing factors for your child's health condition. I approach a child's autism-spectrum condition from a medical standpoint. I want to know what is going on medically.

Do they have nutritional imbalances, yeast or bacterial overgrowth, food allergies and sensitivities, biochemical imbalances and/or immune system dysfunction, and heavy metal toxicity? All these factors can contribute to your child not getting well, and just as importantly contributing to their autism.

Treating the Patient - Not their Diagnosis

As a physician I do not treat autism per se. Instead, I evaluate children medically who suffer with a myriad of health problems such as food intolerances, nutritional deficiencies, heavy metal toxins, viral, yeast, parasitic and bacterial infections – all who happen to have a diagnosis of an autism-spectrum disorder. In the course of treating their medical condition, like any doctor would do for their patient, a child's autism often gets better, and sometimes completely goes away. Speech, eye contact, attention, focusing, language, socialization and more are things that can be improved by addressing the underlying medical issues of a child. It really is not a big mystery to evaluate them medically. The problem is most of the medical community doesn't bother to look or believe that medical problems exist or medical treatment is even indicated. It is assumed by most medical authorities that many kids with autism have digestive problems or it is common for them to have repeated ear infections. This is nonsense! These kids need to be evaluated medically and treated if abnormalities are found.

Your Child Deserves Better

In my experience, the traditional medical community is ill-equipped to evaluate autism-spectrum children and provide them with well-rounded treatment options beyond just some cursory medications to control behavior. This is why working with a clinician trained in the various biomedical therapies is essential. Your doctor has to be open-minded to all aspects of evaluation, therapies and healing. There are no quick fixes, magic creams or potions that will make your child's autism go away. Persistence, hard-work and dedication are essential, but miracles can and do happen!

There are no guarantees of absolute recovery for all children on the spectrum. Yes, some do. However, what is more common is that they become healthier, more social, and more engaged with their family and peers.

My Comprehensive Biomedical Approach to Testing and Treatment for a Child with ASD – various scenarios of intervention, diagnostic findings, and patient responses.

Over the next few pages I am going to describe in more detail how I approach children on the spectrum and what I have commonly seen in clinical practice. Along with these descriptions will be brief cases of children who highlight the various biomedical issues – food sensitivities including gluten and casein, heavy metal toxicity, digestive problems including yeast, bacteria and parasites, and more.

If we take the above list of characteristics for a regressive ASD child (non-regressive ASD can apply to the following discussion as well) and begin to evaluate them medically we can see many of the typical medical problems become revealed.

A Comprehensive Laboratory Assessment:

Listed below are the common laboratory tests that I perform. Of course, not all tests are needed for all kids, but the bulk of children eventually need many of these tests:

- Organic Acid Test
- Comprehensive Stool Analysis w/parasitological testing
- Comprehensive Food Sensitivity Profile (IgG)
- Urinary Peptides
- Hair Analysis
- Fecal Metal Analysis
- Packed Red Blood Cell Analysis (mineral assessment)
- Immunoglobulins: Total IgG, IgM, IgA, IgE

- Comprehensive Blood Chemistry including liver & kidney function, electrolytes, serum iron & ferritin, thyroid panel: TSH, free T4 and T3, blood fats: total cholesterol, HDL, LDL, and homocysteine.
- Viral panel – IgG & IgM: EBV, CMV, Herpes I, II, VI, Varicella, as well as Measles and Rubella IgG, as well as Natural Killer (NK) Cell Analysis and Activity.
- ANA, C-Reactive Protein, Sed Rate
- Porphyrin Profile
- Streptococcus Panel: ASO titer (anti-streptolysin O) and Anti-DNAse B – both are helpful in cases of recurrent infections, i.e. tonsils, throat as well as OCD, Tics, and Tourette's.
- Plasma Amino Acids
- Other Labs of Interest that are commonly helpful:

  - Borrelia bacteria (Lyme Disease) and co-infection analysis
  - DPP-IV antibodies
  - Gliadin Antibodies & Anti-transglutaminase (celiac disease)
  - Helicobacter pylori – stool antigen and IgG, IgM, IgA
  - Folate Receptor Antibodies

NOTE: There are other lab tests that can be done, but the list above is quite extensive.

Test Highlight (Organic Acid Test):

The organic acid test is essential to analyze for yeast, and bacterial overgrowth – including clostridium. It is also helpful to assess the level of oxalate excretion, and other factor's related to glutathione and antioxidant status, serotonin

16

metabolism, quinolinic acid production (a marker for potential brain toxicity reaction) as well as markers for in-born errors of metabolism including oxalate and amino acid dysfunction.

Case #1: Yeast and Pervasive Developmental Disorder (PDD)

Mark was one of my first ASD cases back in 1998. He was a 2 year old boy diagnosed with PPD-NOS (not otherwise specified). His development was typical of the history listed above. Multiple ear infections had led to repeated antibiotics for months on end. Loose stools were the norm as he struggled to maintain eye contact and learn in school. I ordered an Organic Acid Test (OAT) from Great Plains laboratory and discovered a massive amount of yeast metabolites – arabinose being the most common and quite elevated in Mark. Being new to biomedicine for autism all I knew to do at the time was make a recommendation for a gluten/casein-free diet and anti-fungal therapy. The anti-fungal medication was called Nystatin. Mark's mother also implemented some basic supplements including a multi-vitamin and mineral, probiotics, and digestive enzymes.

After 18 months of continuous use of Nystatin, dietary modification and general nutritional support Mark was mainstreamed into regular school and continued to do well. His repeat OAT finally showed no yeast overgrowth. This case illustrated for me the powerful changes that could happen for an ASD child with basic dietary intervention and prolonged anti-fungal therapy.

Yeast has a tremendous ill-effect on health. What are common in children with yeast overgrowth are behaviors that suggest dissociation, withdraw, and aloofness. The most common behaviors are the following:

- Poor eye contact
- Increased self-stimulatory behavior – fixating on spinning objects, odd hand movements including and finger-flicking in front of eyes.
- Toe-walking
- Becoming withdrawn
- "Silly, goofy and/or giddy" – but this is not a behavior that involves other people. The child becomes silly, goofy and/or giddy to themselves. Parents will often describe that their child appears drunk.
- Increased sugar craving
- Increased desire to masturbate
- Overall increased sensory seeking behavior, i.e. pressure

Other parents can describe other more subtle differences, but those listed above are fairly common manifestations. What is most common with "yeasty" behavior is a *giddiness* that overcomes a child as though they are drugged or drunk. When they are put on medications such as Nystatin or natural remedies such as oregano oil and/or grapefruit seed extract these behaviors improve. However, another common bug detected on the OAT test from Great Plains Laboratory can give quite the opposite pattern – its name is Clostridia.

Clostridia – and the Case of Violent Behavior

Clostridia is an anaerobic (doesn't thrive in an oxygen rich environment) bacteria that invades the intestines of susceptible individuals. The most commonly discussed clostridia bacteria, particularly in hospital settings, is Clostridium difficle. This organism is a major problem as it has developed resistance to common antibiotics. Ironically, Clostridium difficle can become an issue in people who have taken long-term antibiotics for infections. In its severe form it can trigger a serious inflammatory bowel condition called pseudomembranous colitis (1). However, there are other species of clostridia that can be problematic without causing this life threatening condition.

The OAT (from Great Plains Laboratory) reveals a specific marker called HPHPA. When this is elevated, the presence of clostridia is defined. The type of clostridia is not specifically isolated, but you will know it is present in your child's digestive system because of the elevated HPHPA marker (2). Unlike yeast overgrowth which can cause the classic "goofy and giddiness" behavior, clostridia can trigger the exact opposite.

Case #2: A Contributor to Aggressive Behavior

Frank was a five year old ASD boy. His history included multiple antibiotics for ear infections over the previous three years. Shortly after a recent upper respiratory infection he started to become more aggressive – hitting, kicking, and screaming. This went on for a few months. The parents began to implement a GF/CF diet which seemed to calm down his behaviors to some degree. They also used some herbal remedies of grapefruit seed extract and caprylic acid. This helped with some of his eye contact issues and focusing capacity. However, Frank was still prone to excessive outbursts – including head banging.

An OAT revealed very high levels of HPHPA. His yeast marker for arabinose was slightly elevated too, and a urinary peptide test was elevated for both gluten and casein. In some kids the HPHPA level may only be slightly elevated -- around 150 to 250. In these situations the use of Culturelle (acidophilus GG) may be effective. However, in Frank's case his HPHPA was over 700! The use of grapefruit seed extract and caprylic helped slightly with his eye contact and focusing, but it was not enough to touch his clostridia problem. Also, implementing the GF/CF diet certainly was beneficial because of his elevated peptides. Ultimately though, he needed more aggressive therapy to lower the clostridia levels.

I implemented a 10 day course of Flagyl (antibiotic) at 40mg/kg – split dosed 3x/day along with Culturelle (Lactobaccilus GG) replenishment at 3 capsules per day for 2 weeks following the Flagyl, and then 2 capsules per day thereafter. This was enough to eradicate the clostridia and keep it from returning. After five days of taking the medication, Frank became non-aggressive, and his tantrums had diminished as well. Within three weeks of completing the therapy, he was much happier, less irritable, and doing well in school again. His head-banging had stopped.

Impact Food Can Have On Behaviors

The idea that food can have an adverse effect on behaviors in children is nothing new. It has been known for years in the biomedical community that peptides from gluten and casein affect certain ASD children (3) as to their behavior and overall cognitive function. These food proteins can also have an adverse affect on immune function as well (4). Also, food coloring and dyes (based on the concept of phenol sensitivity), and certain substances such as salicylates (Feingold institute - www.feingold.org) all can contribute to adverse behaviors such as aggression, hyperactivity, lack of focus and more (5).

The Organic Acid Test along with the Urinary Peptide and Comprehensive Food IgG profile (all from Great Plains Laboratory) gives more evidence of food sensitivities and the usefulness of implementing various dietary therapies – including the Gluten & Casein-free diet, the Specific Carbohydrate Diet (SCD) and/or the Low Oxalate Diet (LOD). At times it is necessary to explore various diets to see which one works best.

Dietary intervention is not always a one size fits all approach. Remember, your child is an individual and their response to a dietary change may be entirely different than another child. When it comes to dietary modifications you will never know the full benefit they can have on your child's health and behavior until you give one of them a try.

The next case is typical of the need for some parents to implement dietary changes in stages. The various tests just mentioned can be helpful if elevations are seen in gluten and/or casein markers, as well as oxalate levels. However, please be advised that the lack of positive finding on a test does not 100% indicate that a sensitivity to food is not an issue, and that benefit could not be achieved with dietary implementation.

Case #3: Self-Injury Behavior (SIB)

– A Complex Case

Derrick was an eight year old boy who was diagnosed at the age of two with "classic" autism. His main issues included SIB (self-injury behavior), aggression, and sleep disorder – he could literally be up through the night for hours. His worst behaviors would many times manifest for one to two hours after school. Other concerns were his lack of speech, self-limited diet (high dairy and grains), and very poor socialization. One curious condition was his very high pain tolerance.

After running an OAT and Urinary Peptide it was determined that Derrick was a child with massive amounts of yeast and clostridia bacteria toxins.

His toxin levels for yeast and bacteria were some of the highest I have ever seen at that time, with his clostridia marker (HPHPA) well over a 1000! Also, his peptide values were elevated as well. The first order of business was to implement some basic supplements including a multi-vitamin, mineral and antioxidants. I also recommended that the parents start the Gluten/Casein-Free Diet.

Because of his severe combativeness the parents had a difficult time getting him to take supplements consistently. However, he was able to take melatonin – 1 mg before bed which helped significantly with sleep. Because of his very high clostridia (HPHPA) and yeast (arabinose) we tried to implement the Flagyl and Diflucan (antifungal).

Unfortunately, because of excessive die-off reactions (die-off is a condition where a child's symptoms worsen because of the toxins being released by eradicating bacteria and yeast) he became even more aggressive and the SIB worsened – this was too much for the parents to handle. Instead, we started him on Culturelle – 1 capsule twice daily and a multi-flora probiotic supplement knowing that in the future we would again need to address the clostridium and yeast. Knowing that severe yeast and bacterial overgrowth problems can thrive in a gut with lots of inflammation we decided to implement the Specific Carbohydrate Diet (SCD).

This diet is based on the work of the late Elaine Gottschall, author of the books "Food and the Gut Reaction" and "Breaking the Vicious Cycle." The premise is individuals with inflammatory bowel diseases such as Crohn's Disease and Ulcerative Colitis have difficulty digesting complex sugars called disaccharides – such as rice, corn and other grain products. This diet has been successful in many children on the autism-spectrum particularly those with

digestive problems such as severe constipation or chronic loose stools – many of these kids eventually get diagnosed with inflammatory bowel disease.

The remarkable thing with Derrick was 5 weeks after starting the SCD, his SIB was virtually gone. Derrick was also taking a medication called Naltrexone 25mg. This medication is used for narcotic addiction – particularly to heroin and morphine. It has been used with success for aggression and SIB in autism. For Derrick, after 5 weeks on the specific carbohydrate diet he no longer needed Naltrexone.

NOTE: Approximately, 3 months into the SCD Derrick began to have some aggressive and self-injury behavior return, but to a much reduced degree than before. He was manageable and did not need medication. The next phase in dietary therapy for him was to implement the Low Oxalate Diet (LOD). The LOD is another dietary intervention that can make a tremendous difference for children on the spectrum.

Oxalates (Oxalic Acid and the Low Oxalate Diet, aka. LOD)

Oxalates are organic compounds found in many grains and vegetables. Because of the overuse of antibiotics and depletion of normal intestinal bacteria which normally degrades oxalates commonly found in our diet, these oxalates (in susceptible individuals) can absorb into the body and form oxalate crystals with various minerals, i.e. calcium-oxalate kidney stones. Much of the research into oxalate problems has been with patients suffering from kidney stones, women with a vaginal pain condition called Vulvadynia (6), and the less common genetic disorders for oxalate metabolism. Susan Owens, an independent biomedical researcher, has introduced the concept and principles of oxalate problems in autistic children and the benefits that can be derived from a low oxalate diet (LOD). William Shaw, Ph.D (of Great Plains Laboratory) has provided research about the problems of oxalates and autism.

With respects to Case #3 (Derrick: Self-Injury Behavior) we began to introduce some basics of the LOD program including calcium/magnesium citrate before meals, and a particular high dose probiotic called VSL#3. Again, within a short period his behavior began to improve. He is an example of a severely autistic child who had significant improvement by implementing some specialized dietary changes. Derrick would not be classified as cured or recovered from autism, but his aggressive and self-abusive behaviors were markedly improved so that he became a more functional member of his family which allowed for some normalcy within the household.

Test Highlight: (Comprehensive Stool Testing)

I cannot emphasize enough the importance of evaluating your child's digestive system as thoroughly as possible. The organic acid test is essential in my laboratory work-up because of its ability to evaluate for various metabolic toxins - from yeast and bacteria, i.e. clostridia. However, the OAT cannot specifically detect for other types of intestinal pathogens such as various opportunistic bacteria (Klebsiella, Pseudomonas, or Citrobacter), as well as parasites such as Blastocystis hominis, Cryptosporidium parvum, Entamoeba histolytica, and Giardia lamblia. These pathogens, especially the parasitic infections, are more common than you think and will never be fully appreciated unless tested for and detected on stool sampling.

When it comes to testing, one of my rules as a physician, especially with respect to digestive system evaluation, is to not be fooled by a lack of digestive symptoms such as diarrhea, constipation, bloating, and excessive gas. I have seen many kids who are loaded with intestinal infections that have no or very little intestinal symptoms.

The lack of these symptoms does not mean everything is okay in your child's gut. You need to do stool testing to make sure everything is fine. I realize there are times when it is extremely difficult to get a stool sample, but in most it is fairly easy to get – gross I know, but manageable.

Parasitic infections are quite common. One in particular is Giardia, also known as the cause of "beaver fever" because it is prevalent in lakes, streams and rivers (7). It can rapidly multiply in the intestinal system causing profound diarrhea and fluid loss. However, Giardia can also become a chronic infection leading to marked food maldigestion (poor digestion). Cats and dogs can harbor giardia and be a reservoir for infection. So can other family members.

Cryptosporidium parvum is another common parasite seen in kids (8). Although it is commonly described as a self-limiting infection, massive infections can be life-threatening. Day care centers are a common place to pick-up cryptosporidium. I have seen patients who never got rid of their original cryptosporidium infection and the organism has become a chronic inhabitant in their intestinal system. Prolonged cryptosporidium can also lead to maldigestion as well.

Entamoeba histolytica is a serious amoeba parasite that can become life-threatening in a susceptible host (9). E. histolytica can take up shop in the gut creating an avenue for yeast overgrowth and maldigestion, or be transported to the liver where it can create abscess formation. E. histolytica is a parasite that should absolutely be eradicated with antibiotics (in my opinion) such as Flagyl, Tinidazole, or Alinia (or other suitable antibiotics) to prevent any recurrence.

In addition to the pathogen examination the Comprehensive Digestive Stool Analysis also provides other useful information regarding digestive system health, such as markers of inflammation, maldigestion and intestinal immune function. The sensitivity testing for specific therapeutic agents such as antibiotic and herbal remedies against common bacteria and yeast organisms are also useful to fine tune treatment programs. However, when it comes to parasitic infections you are commonly left with using medications that are known to eradicate a broad spectrum of these bugs. This was the case with Eric who had some profound changes after treating for parasites.

Case #4: An Explosion of Language

Eric was a 5 year old ASD child who suffered from severe constipation, bloating, gas and obvious discomfort from a lack of normal bowel function. He also had significant language delays and struggled to speak appropriately for his age. A myriad of labs were performed including parasitology testing which revealed a chronic cryptosporidium infection. It was hard to know how long he had been harboring this parasite in his gut, but it was clearly a long-time. I was also suspicious of possible worm infections – roundworm being most common – but had no direct evidence of this. Worm infections like roundworm and pinworms can be a cause of constipation. We decided to implement a treatment course of Alinia (Nitazoxanide) 200mg – one dose twice daily for 3 days, wait 7 days and repeat. The following day and for the next week Eric's speech exploded. As his mother described when Eric was in his speech therapy session the instructor could not get a word in edge wise. Eventually, Eric needed further intestinal evaluation and therapy, but the major instigating factor for his progress in speech was eradicating intestinal parasites and the release of backed up stool.

Test Highlight (Heavy Metal Assessment)

Heavy metal exposure is quite prevalent in our modern world. All around us are manufactured products that have heavy metals like antimony and tin that we use in our homes, cars, offices, schools. We are all exposed to these toxins and no one can avoid them 100% of the time. Unfortunately, we do not live in a metal free bubble. When it comes to autism we know heavy metal exposure is a risk factor for these children.

Diagnostic assessments have been done that prove the existence of toxic levels of heavy metals in children with autism compared to neurotypical kids (10). In the next few sections we will explore some issues with respect to heavy metal toxicity and an example of heavy metal detoxification therapy. What is important to understand is that various heavy metals tests have different usefulness.

Fecal Metals

I will commonly use the fecal metal (stool) test as a marker for environmental exposure to heavy metals. Because the stool is a reflection of what has been taken into the body via food, air (swallowed air), and water it helps to detail contamination. The fecal metal test should not be used as the sole indicator of detoxifying metals from within the body, but it is possible to see elevated levels of heavy metals on a stool sample that overtime could reflect dumping of internal toxins into the gut.

However, my preference is to use fecal metal testing as a baseline evaluation to assess a child's environment to see if there is anything excessive that a child is being exposed to. I do not expect to see absolute zeros for each heavy metal tested because all of us are exposed to environmental pollutants. Instead, I use the fecal metals test to isolate certain metals that come back very elevated like mercury, lead, arsenic and even antimony.

Case #5 is an example of the usefulness of fecal metal testing, especially with respect to in-home heavy metals exposure. When it comes to biomedical assessment a lot has been mentioned about mercury exposure and toxicity, but many times there are other heavy metals as well.

Case #5 – Antimony On The Rise

John was a three year old boy brought to me for heavy metal assessment. His parents concerns were heavy metal exposure after a hair analysis showed elevated antimony. We ordered a fecal metal test. The test reported extremely high levels of antimony. Not knowing the source, but suspecting it was coming from within the child's home, his parents hired an environmental home inspector. What came back was nothing short of amazing. The home inspector had taken a sample of the carpet padding and had it analyzed for heavy metals. The results showed that the antimony level was 150x what was considered safe by the Environmental Protection Agency (EPA). The parents had the padding replaced and the exposure problem was solved.

What was interesting was that the parents were tested for antimony on hair and fecal sampling also and their levels were much less than John's. Why would this be? I surmised as a three year old who spends most of his day close to the carpet he was exposed to higher amounts of antimony dust being kicked into the air – probably no more than 12 to 18 inches - just the perfect level for John to inhale and swallow.

Manufactured antimony is commonly used as a fire retardant material in baby clothes, cribs, and mattresses. It is also found in upholstery, paints, ceramic tile, carpet, plastic toys, and even water bottles.

Hair Analysis

A hair analysis is an inexpensive, easy to perform assessment of heavy metal exposure. It gives a picture of what your child has been exposed to and what they may be excreting through their hair. A hair analysis also gives a snapshot picture of mineral levels as well. Although, technically a hair mineral level is not going to give absolute indicators of all mineral levels found in the blood stream – minerals such as cobalt, iodine, lithium, and selenium are fairly close to what is seen on blood testing.

Blood Metal Testing

If you look at blood testing such as found in the Red Blood Cell Analysis (RBC Metals) it will indicate intracellular levels of essential minerals – an important test for assessing minerals. However, it does not answer all the questions concerning heavy metal toxicity. Generally, blood tests for heavy metals such as lead and mercury are the best indicators of recent or ongoing exposure, but not past exposure where the metals have been lodged in different body tissue such as the brain.

Urine Metal Testing

The urine test is commonly used to assess what is being excreted out of the body while undergoing heavy metal detoxification (chelation) therapy. The toxic urine test (urine metals) is a valuable tool and helps track metal excretion overtime. However, it only indicates what is coming out of your child's body – not how much is left behind.

In fact, there is no one heavy metal test that gives absolute levels of heavy metals such as mercury or lead. You must use a variety of heavy metal tests, along with clinical suspicion and the willingness to implement detoxification therapy to see what type of clinical response is achieved. However, there is one test profile that has shown to be an indicator of toxicity to heavy metals. Again, it does not give absolute levels of heavy metals, but instead it provides what I call the "toxic effect" of heavy metals at the cellular level in the body. This test is called the Porphyrin Profile.

Porphyrin Profile

Porphyrins are chemical byproducts of heme production. Heme is an essential chemical in our body that produces hemoglobin (carries oxygen to all the cells of the body). Heme also functions inside our cells for energy production, and in the liver for detoxification support.

Heme is also responsible for helping to rid the brain of a substance called beta-amyloid which is associated with Alzheimer's Disease. With respect to autism and the discussion about heavy metal toxicity the porphyrin profile is very useful. It turns out that various steps in the biochemical factory line to produce heme are adversely affected by heavy metals such as mercury, lead, arsenic, tin, and others (11).

As mentioned, the usefulness of this profile is to get a better idea of cellular toxicity (what is happening inside the cell) with respects to heavy metal exposure. Heme is produced via mechanisms attached to our cells mitochondria (which produce a lot of cell energy chemicals), and if metals are present in significant quantities they can disrupt mitochondrial production of heme. Therefore, various porphyrin markers will likely be elevated. Case #6 describes a typical case of heavy metal toxicity and the need to implement detoxification therapy.

Case #6 – The Importance of Heavy Metal Detoxification

Jake was a typical ASD child. He had fairly normal development until he was about 15 months old. He had language deficits typical of many kids on the spectrum that manifested around this age. The parents in retrospect felt that he started to show some lack of progress in speech even earlier, as well as eye contact, but overall nothing too alarming. He was still playful, inquisitive, and generally a happy thriving child. It wasn't until after his 15 month vaccines did things start to change drastically for Jake. His eye contact began to rapidly disappear, language was lost, and odd behaviors became manifest such as obsession with spinning objects, increased sound and touch sensitivity, and increased isolation.

Being a child born in the late 90's, it was clear his vaccine schedule was high in vaccines containing Thimerosal (mercury preservative). Other potential exposures were his mother's amalgam (mercury fillings) which could have led to in-utero exposure, and other environmental sources. Whatever the source of exposure, it was clear, based on heavy metal assessment that Jake was a candidate for heavy metal detoxification. By implementing heavy metal detoxification therapy using DMPS (a specific medication for the removal of heavy metals like mercury) as well as vitamin, mineral, and antioxidant support Jake began to make progress. His improvement was slow and steady – like it commonly is with heavy metal detoxification – but eventually his issues of spinning and sound sensitivity were reduced. He had better eye contact, as well as more sophisticated speech and improved cognitive function.

For Jake, as with many of children on the autism-spectrum, heavy metal detoxification is an essential medical treatment.

There are many options available for biomedical therapies. Each child needs to be assessed individually. Through history evaluation, diagnostic testing, and therapy implementation many children will reveal their underlying biomedical issues – which sometimes are not the same for every child. To say that all autism is caused by any one thing is too simplistic. In my opinion there is no doubt that heavy metals such as mercury play a significant role, but so do immune system imbalances, methylation defects, etc. In the near future we will likely see autism not described as one single entity, but instead looked at as different types of autism, or as David Kirby states (author of Evidence of Harm) – "autisms." The list below describes other considerations for children on the autism-spectrum. Testing is available for many of these scenarios and various therapies can be helpful:

- Viral Issues – including herpes infections. Many children have responded well to various antiviral therapies including Valtrex, acyclovir or herbal remedies such as Larrea tridentata, Samento, as well as Lauricidin.

- Natural Killer (NK) Cell Activity deficiency and autoimmunity. A major regulator over cell-mediated immune function and its role in preventing and eradicating viral infections, NK activity can be enhanced by therapeutic Transfer Factor. Clearly, immune modulating therapy is necessary for some children on the autism-spectrum who tend to show imbalances in immune function. Immune dysfunction of NK Cells and other immune factors can lead to brain inflammation through a mechanism called microglia activation.
- Streptococcus infection and OCD (obsessive compulsive behavior) – a medical condition called PANDAS is a known as neuropsychiatric condition triggered by streptococcal bacteria. Transfer factor, immune therapy called intravenous immunoglobulin therapy (IVIG), and certain antibiotics may be helpful in alleviating this condition.

- Lyme Disease or Borrelia-Related Complex (Borrelia infection without an obvious tick-bite exposure). When it comes to autism or other types of chronic neurological conditions, these infectious entities can be an issue. Borrelia burgdefori (the causative organism for Lyme Disease) is no exception (12). Antibiotics, as well as herbal therapies can be used with good success.

Finally, three very important therapies which were not illustrated in the case reports above, but are essential factors in helping children on the autism-spectrum are Methyl-B12 (methylcobalamin) therapy, Hyperbaric Oxygen Therapy (HBOT), and Respen-A therapy. The methyl-B12 therapy is at the cornerstone of supporting detoxification and normal function of the methylation biochemistry for children on the autism-spectrum (13). HBOT plays a significant role in reducing neurological inflammation, promoting increased oxygen uptake into the brain, and overall cognitive improvement (14), and finally Respen-A plays a role in helping serotonin metabolism which is critical for improved cognition, mood, socialization, and improved language.

References:

(1) Bartlett JG: Pseudomembranous enterocolitis and antibiotic-associated colitis. In: Feldman M, Scharschmidt BF, Sleisenger MH, eds. Sleisenger and Fordtran's Gastrointestinal and Liver Disease. 6th ed. Philadelphia, Pa: WB Saunders Co; 1998: 1633-1647.

(2) Elsden S et al. The end products of the metabolism of aromatic amino acids by clostridia. 1976 Arch Microbiol 107: 283-8.

(3) Reichelt KL and Kvisbery A-M. Why diet is useful in some autistic children: results so far. Presentation at DAN! Portland Conference, 2003: DAN! Fall 2003 Syllabus 91-99.

(4) Vodjani A, Pangborn JB et al. Infections, toxic chemicals and dietary peptides binding to lymphocyte receptors and tissue enzymes are major instigators of autoimmunity in autism Int.J.Immunopath and Pharmacol 16 no.3 (2003) 189-199.

(5) Rowe K.S. Synthetic food coloring and hyperactivity: A double-blind crossover study. 1998 Aust Paediatr J 24: 143-47.

(6) Sarma AV et al. Epidemiology of Vulvar Vestibulitis Syndrome: an exploratory case-control study. Sex Transm Infect. 1999 Oct, 75(5): 320-6.

(7) Centers for Disease Control – Division of Parasitic Infections (http://www.cdc.gov/ncidod/dpd/parasites/giardiasis/factsht_giardia.htm).

(8) Center for Disease Control – Division of Parasitic Infections (http://www.cdc.gov/ncidod/dpd/parasites/cryptosporidiosis/factsht_cryptosporidiosis.htm).

(9) Centers for Disease Control – Division of Parasitic Infections (http://www.cdc.gov/ncidod/dpd/parasites/amebiasis/factsht_amebiasis.htm).

(10) Woods JS, Martin MD, Naleway CA, Echeverria D. Urinary porphyrin profiles as a biomarker of mercury exposure: studies on dentists with occupational exposure to mercury vapor. J Toxicol Environ Health. 1993 Oct-Nov; 40(2-3):235-46.

(11) Nataf R, Skorupka C, Amet L, Lam A, Springbett A, Lathe R. Porphyrinuria in childhood autistic disorder: implications for environmental toxicity. Toxicol Appl Pharmacol. 2006 Jul 15; 214(2):99-108.

(12) American College of Physicians. Guidelines for laboratory evaluation in the diagnosis of Lyme's disease. Ann Intern Med. 1997.

(13) James J, Cutler P, Neubrander J, et al. Metabolic biomarkers of increased oxidative stress and impaired methylation capacity in children with autism. Am J Clin Nutr. 2004; 80:1611-7.

(14) Rossingol DA, Small T. Hyperbaric Oxygen Therapy Improves Symptoms in Autistic Children. Medical Veritas 3 (2006) 1-4.

Chapter 2

Biomedicine as a Treatment Option for Individuals with an Autism-Spectrum Disorder

The Roots of Biomedical Therapy for Autism

The biomedical movement for autism-spectrum disorders got its birth from an organization called the Autism Research Institute (ARI) founded by Bernard Rimland, Ph.D in San Diego, CA. Dr. Rimland, even from the early days of autism awareness, felt that autism had roots in biological causation, and was not just a psychological disorder. Dr. Rimland advocated the use of vitamin B6 and magnesium which his research showed helped with cognitive function for autistic individuals. Based on his progressive research and collaboration with like-minded physicians who were using nutrition and targeted vitamin and mineral therapies for their chronically ill patients, including individuals with autism, the Defeat Autism Now! organization was born. From their original meetings has sprung forth a highly respected group of clinicians and researchers dedicated to treating the various health issues seen so commonly in autistic individuals.

The ARI is to be commended for their ongoing dedication to helping unravel the health issues of people with an autism-spectrum disorder. Their conferences are held twice yearly and are an incredible resource of information for parents and doctors seeking answers about biomedical intervention. Of course, the concepts of good diet, proper immune and digestive function that promote health and vitality are nothing new to the world of natural medicine.

Natural healers, herbalists and nutritional laymen have for years been promoting healthy diets and the removal of toxins for disease prevention. However, what the Autism Research Institute has been able to do is bring these issues to the forefront of the autism epidemic which we now face. In a sea of ignorance from which most of the medical community still exists with respect to treatment for your autistic loved one, the Autism Research Institute has now bridged that gap and is making it known that biomedical therapies are a viable option for parents and/or care-givers for someone with autism.

Basic Overview of Biomedicine for Autism

- More than just a psychological or neurodevelopmental condition.

- Belief that the majority of autistic-spectrum children (as well as teenagers and adults) are dealing with underlying biological and toxicity disorder.

- Includes children with attention-deficit (ADD) and attention deficit hyperactivity disorder (ADHD).

- Includes children with other neurodevelopmental problems.

- Heavy metals, food sensitivities, nutritional deficiencies, chronic infections, immune dysfunction and genetic susceptibilities are at the core of their health problems.

- Biological problems involving the brain, immune, digestive, hormone and biochemical systems.

- Totally false that there is no hope for recovery.

In understanding this paradigm it should become evident to the rest of the medical community that autism no longer should be described as purely a brain disorder, but instead a multi-system disorder involving the digestive, biochemical, detoxification, digestive, and metabolic systems that affect the brain.

It is my belief that a biomedical approach is ABSOLUTELY necessary for children (teenagers and adults) if recovery is desired. This is not to say that every person will reach the same level of improvement or that every child is recoverable. Recovery to the point of being indistinguishable from a neurotypical child or adult is an individual matter. However, doing everything we can to improve the health potential of your loved one is certainly within the realm of possibility.

Every parent wants to see their child reach their full potential. There are many different faces of autism, and certainly many different degrees of autism-spectrum severity. The point is that not everyone is recoverable from their particular health condition. Not every person who has cancer will survive, or who suffers a heart attack will live. Medicine does not have 100% guarantees for any treatment it has to offer for any illness. Life just doesn't work this way. However, this does not mean we don't try and do something about these illnesses to the best of our abilities.

As a society, and certainly as a medical community, we do everything we can to try and improve the health condition of our population – at least this is what should happen. So too, the biomedical approach does not offer guarantees for absolute recovery. However, there are many individuals who will improve their overall health and mental/emotional condition to the point of being contributing members to society (if not just their own family which is incredibly important).

Optimizing Potential

My approach for *all* patients is to optimize their health potential. Being a father of two children I want the best for them for whatever capacity they have in this life. Some things I can control and some things I cannot. So too, you as a parent hold the keys to your child's success. The more doors you can open for them the better chance they have to be able to function effectively in society.

With respects to biomedical therapies you can help to open up those doors with diet and nutritional supplements, detoxification treatment and other complementary therapies. There are many choices and a wide array of options. The more doors you open simultaneously the better their chances of improved health. The only thing we do not have control over is your child's response to various biomedical therapies. Once again we are left up to the nature of the individual, in this case your child, to determine for us their overall response and improvement.

The Puzzle Scenario

There are many questions to be answered regarding the cause and treatment of autism. The solutions are not always simple, the cause is often multi-factorial, and the testing and subsequent treatments sometimes complicated and expensive. It is important to realize that with everything in medicine there are no guarantees of absolute illness recovery, especially with complex disorders involving the nervous system. However, there is reason for hope and enthusiasm.

Your child is like a puzzle. The factors which influence their physical health and mental/emotional well-being are many. Your child may be more prone to frequent colds and allergies; whereas another child may suffer with chronic digestive problems. They may have a food fixation with an extremely limited diet; whereas another child may eat everything in sight - including their steamed broccoli and carrots (which is a rarity even in my house with my kids!). Every person is unique and they need to be understood this way. Taking this into consideration also creates some difficulties with respects to biomedical therapy because your child may not respond very well to a certain therapies such as Methyl-B12 (which is rare!); whereas another child starts speaking in sentences almost immediately - hence, the puzzle scenario.

A parent in my practice described the puzzle scenario this way, "You do not know if your child is a 6 piece, a 60 piece, or a 600 piece puzzle. You have to keep trying different puzzle pieces to see what will work for them." I could not agree more. This same scenario applies to non-biomedical therapy as well. Some kids do real well with Applied Behavior Analysis (ABA therapy) while others progress significantly with speech or occupational therapies. Many times it is the simultaneous application of various pieces that make your child's puzzle come together.

Dietary changes, nutritional supplementation, laboratory testing, and the other therapeutic biomedical options including heavy metal chelation (detoxification), methylcobalamin therapy (injections, intranasal), immune support, Respen-A, and others are many times recommended. I have adapted my approach from a number of different styles including the Defeat Autism Now! programs, Dr. Yasko's genetic profiling and supplementation programs; herbal traditions of Dr. John Ray Christopher, Functional Diagnostic Medicine and BioHealth intervention of the brilliant William Timmins, N.D., the osteopathic philosophy of James Jealous, D.O. and more. Every doctor or health practitioner learns from their predecessors in their respective field of medicine. The biomedical movement for autism is no different. There is a tremendous amount we know about the causative factors behind the autistic condition, but there is also a lot more to learn. I do not have all the answers to this complex problem (but, I do have access to a wealth of knowledgeable individuals and resources for research and cutting edge information), nor does anyone else, but I hope at least the information and outline I provide in this book will serve as a useful mechanism for you to help save your child now.

The Biomedical Approach – Incorporates Many Aspects of Medicine

A biomedical approach utilizes a wide variety of therapies, testing and at times medication (if needed). Listed below is a brief outline:

Diagnostic Testing

- o Hair – heavy metals, nutrients
- o Urine – heavy metals, porphyrin analysis, peptides (fragments of gluten and casein), nutrients, amino acids, byproducts of yeast and bacteria
- o Blood – heavy metals, nutrients, amino acids, immune markers, biotoxins such as mold, Lyme, blood chemistry, thyroid, liver and kidney function assessment, viruses, bacteria, etc.
- o Stool (Fecal) – heavy metals, bacteria, yeast (candida), parasites, digestive function markers, such as inflammation and enzyme function

- **Medications (when necessary)**
  - o Anti-fungal (Nystatin, Diflucan, etc.)
  - o Antiviral (Famvir, Valtrex, Zovirax, etc.)
  - o Antibacterial/Parasites (Flagyl, Vancomycin, Alinia, Zithromax, etc.)

- **Dietary and Lifestyle Modifications**
  - o Gluten/Casein/Soy-free Diet
  - o GAPS Diet (Gut and Psychology Syndrome Diet)
  - o Body Ecology Diet

- o Specific Carbohydrate Diet
- o Low Oxalate Diet
- o No More Junk Food Diet
- **Nutritional Supplements**
  - o Vitamins, Minerals, Antioxidants, Amino Acids
  - o Specialized Nutrients (B12, DMG, Folinic Acid or Methyl-Folate, Probiotics, etc.)
  - o Herbal and Homeopathic Remedies
- **Additional Therapies**
  - o Far Infra-red Sauna
  - o Heavy Metal Detoxification (DMPS, DMSA, EDTA, natural remedies)
  - o Hyperbaric Oxygen Therapy (HBOT)
  - o Immune Therapy
  - o Methyl-B12 Therapy (injections, nasal, lollipop)
  - o Respen-A (low dose reserpine)
  - o Folinic Acid (high dose for suspected cerebral folate deficiency) – also methyl-folate supplementation
  - o Bioterrain Homeopathic and Spagyric Detoxification Remedies

Biomedical therapy blends well with other non-biomedical therapies such as speech, behavioral and auditory processing therapy.

What is the Bottom Line?

Not everything in the various biomedical protocols, including all the information in this book or my approach, may be necessary to evaluate and treat every autism-spectrum child. Your loved one is unique in their personality and biochemistry. They deserve individual attention in regards to their health and biomedical support.

It is my firm belief that to support the foundation of your child's health will give great improvements in their autism-spectrum condition. By eliminating heavy metal and chemical toxins, opportunistic organisms such as yeast, pathogenic bacteria, parasites and viruses, many times the barriers to your child's healing are removed. This, at times, is hard work and takes persistence and dedication on your part. In the end, the rewards are gratifying and the outcome sometimes miraculous. However, the bottom line to this story is that no one can convince you that a biomedical approach for your autism-spectrum child is worthwhile. You must come to this conclusion yourself.

Chapter 3

Answering an Important Question for Yourself

as a Parent or Caregiver

We closed chapter 2 with the statement "No one can convince you that the biomedical approach for your autism-spectrum child is worthwhile, you must come to this conclusion yourself." This section is meant to invoke in you a response to a very important question. The answer to this question is critical for you as a parent or care-giver when looking to implement biomedical therapy. I do not mean to imply that if you do not or cannot answer this question for yourself at this time that you cannot start a biomedical program. However, ultimately long-term understanding of biomedicine and the success that can be derived from its potential benefits may be compromised if you do not embrace what a biomedical program has to offer.

This is not only a question that I believe needs to be answered by *all* parents seeking biomedical assessment and care, but of doctors and health providers who are looking to venture down this path as well. By the way, this was a question I needed to answer for myself many years ago because it was not inherently clear to me when I first started working with kids on the spectrum as to what was going on in their bodies medically.

Okay, are you ready to answer the question? Or at least look at the question and contemplate an answer? If so, then turn the page.

Do you believe your child's autism-spectrum disorder stems from a toxicity issue (medical problem) and is not just a developmental brain disorder?

What I mean by this is do you feel your child's autism was caused by a reaction to a vaccine, heavy metal poisons, environmental factors from previous harmful exposures as an infant or your exposure before and during pregnancy, or a combination of all of these. Let me clarify one thing. You have already read in this book about the various medical issues related to autism. When I say "toxicity issue" what I mean is a medical issue or condition. Toxicity does not just come from an external toxin like mercury, lead or environmental chemicals. Toxins can be generated by our own metabolism such as the over-production of ammonia, or within the digestive tract from faulty digestion. Toxins can also result from infections such as bacteria, parasite and/or yeast, as well as food toxins (1).

So, again, what was your initial response to the question above?

YES! – turn 1 page over
NO! – turn 2 pages over
You are not sure! – keep reading

Yes!

If you answered "Yes" then your life as a parent or caregiver trying to help your child just got easier, but it also just got more complicated.

Why?

Because any long-term biomedical approach takes a certain amount of dedication, self-education and motivation, persistence and ultimately partnering with a dedicated physician or other health practitioner to help sort through all the pieces to your child's puzzle.

However, your life also just got more interesting, uplifting, and hopeful as you will discover that there are many things to learn with regards to improving the health of your child.

If you answered **NO** to the above question…

No!

Your decisions regarding biomedical interventions are now more difficult.

Why?

Because to fully embrace the biomedical path it takes dedication and persistence to learn what is available and possibly needed to help your child. In short, you have to understand why and how many of the therapies that are available can help. This does not mean you have to become a biochemist or know the intricate details of physiology. In essence, you do not need to know the intricate details of photosynthesis to grow a tree, but you should have some basic knowledge about soil preparation, fertilizers and water requirements if you want your tree to be tall and healthy. So what are your options?

Options:

- Do nothing.
- Do more research about biomedical options and toxicity issues in relationship to autism.
- Implement the basics – supplements such as multi-vitamin and multi minerals, zinc, cod liver oil, gluten and casein-free diet (a better option may be the Specific Carbohydrate Diet if your child suffers from profound intestinal inflammation, i.e. chronic loose stools, swollen abdomen) and see what happens.
- Basically, plant a tree, water it, and see what happens.

In my experience there is nothing harmful or inherently dangerous that has ever occurred by attempting to implement some dietary changes and basic supplements.

As a physician I had to answer these questions for myself. I needed to come to some resolution about what I believed from what I was seeing in the medical literature regarding autism and what I was seeing in my patient population. The answer for me when I finally realized the importance of this question, "Do you believe the root cause of autism-spectrum disorders stems from a toxicity issue?" The answer was a resounding YES!

This is the approach I take. This book, my practice, my health programs and educational material including webinars, articles, biomedical websites such as www.AutismActionPlan.com, and www.AutismRecoveryTreatment.com all revolve around the central aspect of toxicity and the implications this has for children on the autism-spectrum. I know we are all exposed to a variety of toxins in our environment. The central difference between one person becoming ill and another not is dependent upon a number of factors - age, underlying health, genetics, environment, sex, and the exposure dosages and rates over time. There is no doubt that children with autism have a weakened capacity to rid their body of various toxin such as heavy metals and that the age of exposure, sex of the child, and genetic susceptibility determines a lot with respect to their overall health outcome. (2) Toxicity is a real thing.

Bottom Line – Again

"No one can convince you that a biomedical approach for your autism-spectrum child is worthwhile. You must come to this conclusion yourself."

References:

(1) Parracho HM, Bingham MO, Gibson GR, McCartney AL. Differences between the gut microflora of children with autistic spectrum disorders and that of healthy children. *J Med Microbiol.* 2005 Oct;54(Pt 10):987-91.
(2) Kern JK, Jones AM. Evidence of toxicity, oxidative stress, and neuronal insult in autism. *J Toxicol Environ Health B Crit Rev.* 2006 Nov-Dec;9(6):485-99.

Chapter 4

Getting Started

The decision to begin biomedical intervention for your child can be an easy one. It just takes making the commitment to say, "I am going to do something." That something is the most beneficial thing you can do for your child, yourself, and your family. You have to want to make a difference. You have to want to improve the health of your child. You also have to recognize that your child likely has medical issues that are contributing to their autism regardless of what your pediatrician states or the autism "experts" claim. Most importantly, you have to want to take control of your child's future, and ultimately your overall family's health.

At this point I am assuming you have made the decision to say, "Yes, I can do this." Now is the time to start implementing a strategy. This strategy or what I call your "Action Plan" is your outline of things to do – a "To Do List" if you will. This to do list is important to have as it will help you create a list of supplements, therapies, and testing that you would like to try for your child. You see there is no one specific way to treat a child with autism – no one right way for every child. The reason is there are no two children with autism that are exactly alike. A specific therapy like high dose vitamin B6 may work wonders for a few children (1), but for some kids creates problems with over-stimulation and hyperactivity. Conversely, your child may respond beautifully to the gluten and casein-free (GFCF) diet while a neighbor's child with a similar diagnosis sees no benefits – even after prolonged use. Medicine is full of these uncertainties, but luckily in the world of medicine, and certainly in the world of biomedical interventions for autism there are many options at our disposal.

Also, when you look at trends in treatment you begin to see that many of the biomedical treatments available seem to help most children. Vitamins, dietary restrictions such as gluten, casein and soy, Methyl-B12, Respen-A, heavy metal detoxification, Hyperbaric Oxygen Therapy (HBOT), etc. are all available therapies. So, let's get started with devising an action plan for your child. Remember you are the driver. You control the steering wheel for the road we are going to travel. Also, you control the gas pedal that determines how fast you will travel down your chosen road. The only thing you do not control is how quickly or intensely your child will respond to a given therapy and whether that therapy will ultimately lead to biomedical success. Be patient and stay the course.

Getting Informed and Maintaining an Open Mind

The first step along the biomedical journey is to begin informing yourself about the various options available for treatment. This can be a daunting task as the list of options is expanding all the time. However, I have some great news for you. To get started you do not have to know one iota of biochemistry, physiology or even medicine.

Being open-minded means different things to different people. You may consider yourself to be incredibly open-minded when it comes to health care. If you are like me you appreciate many possibilities of healing. This could include traditional medications, supplements, diet, herbs, homeopathy, hands-on therapies such as osteopathy, chiropractic or massage, color and sound therapy, magnets, sauna therapy, hyperbaric oxygen, nature therapy, and prayer. The list could be endless. Or you may be more inclined to believe the "If I cannot see, feel, or taste it, then it doesn't exist" mentality. There is no right or wrong approach. It's an individual thing.

Understanding the 4 Major Categories of Treatment

This section will briefly explain my 4 major categories of treatment when it comes to helping your child.

1. Reducing the Toxic Stress

In this example, stress is considered to be the various toxins from foods, heavy metals and environmental chemicals, and infections that may be affecting your child's body. From my experience the reason we are seeing an epidemic in autism-spectrum disorders is because genetically (more specifically biochemically) these children have a greater susceptibility to having problems eliminating the increasing number of toxins from their bodies compared to neurotypical children.

When considering the issue of reducing toxic stress the first and easiest place to start is in your own home. From chemical cleaners, pesticides, perfumes and colognes, air fresheners and laundry detergent to the food in your kitchen cupboard there are many agents that can affect your child's health. This process can take some time to learn and will require your time and effort to investigate, but often changing a few products you purchase such as natural laundry detergent in place of perfumed artificial detergents, or fresh squeezed juices instead of soda pop can make a nice difference in overall health for a sensitive child.

I always recommend exploring your local health food store or specialty markets for more natural product alternatives. Here are a few suggestions you can implement to lessen the toxic burdens:

- Buy organic fruits and vegetables.
- Buy organic juices.
- Store left-over food in glass containers instead of plastics.
- Do not cook in the microwave, especially with plastic containers.
- Eliminate soda–regular and decaffeinated.
- No caffeine drinks for kids.
- Purchase a home water filtration unit for the entire house.
- If you own a pool replace the chlorinator with a salt water system.
- If not able to swim in chlorine free pools, then bath in epsom salt baths afterwards (usually one to two cups will suffice).
- Epsom salt cream/lotions work well after swimming in chlorine pools as well. New Beginnings carries Epsom Salt Cream – www.nbnus.com.

- No more fast food. Avoid the McDonalds and Burger Kings of the world. You will truly be healthier for it in my opinion.
- Eliminate regular laundry detergent for eco-friendly brands usually purchased from health markets. Most regular detergents are loaded with perfumes and dyes.
- Avoid wearing cologne and perfumes around your child.
- No smoking.
- Start shopping at health food markets, or your local farmers market for the majority of your food and produce. Make sure the bulk of your produce is organic.

A good resource guide for improving the living environment of your home with regards to chemicals and decreasing the unnecessary chemical additives and preservatives in foods and beverages is **"Home Safe Home"** by Debra Lynn Dadd.

2. Reducing Allergy and Inflammation

Toxins in our body will increase the potential for allergy, and allergy generates inflammation. Inflammation is very damaging to your child's body, especially their fragile brain, and especially if the inflammation is chronic. Neurological conditions such as Parkinson's Disease, Alzheimer's and Multiple Sclerosis are all worsened by inflammation.

Neurological inflammation is nothing new to autism research as various studies show a strong correlation between the various cellular mechanism of inflammation and autism. An example is the activation of cells in the brain called neuroglia. Activation of these cells, i.e. through a virus infection can trigger inflammation in the brain (2).

Toxins of many forms such as foods, viruses, bacteria, chemicals, and heavy metals can all generate inflammation. Various biomedical approaches are designed to help reduce these various forms of toxins to alleviate neurological inflammation. You can begin by implementing some basic changes listed below.

One method of reducing allergy symptoms to foods and environmental triggers such as molds, grasses, pollens, etc., is **NAET** (nambudripad's allergy elimination technique – www.naet.com or **BioSet** www.bioset-institute.com. These forms of natural healing utilize homeopathic dilutions of common allergens to reduce allergy sensitivities. I have seen these therapies work well in improving children's health, behavior and well-being. Please see above web links for more information and practitioners in your area who provide these therapies.

Some children are extremely sensitive to allergens in their environment and may require more traditional allergy injections; while others can be relieved by taking seasonal allergy medications like Zyrtec or Singulair. In less sensitive kids an alternative to these medications are common herbal remedies such as stinging nettles, or plant based substances such as quercetin and/or bromelain. New Beginnings Nutritionals carries a product called A&I Formula which is a natural remedy for environmental allergy – www.nbnus.com.

Other options are the specific diets such as the Gluten/Casein-free diet (soy-free is best as well), Specific Carbohydrate Diet

(SCD), Low Oxalate Diet (LOD) and Feingold diet. Chapter 8 discusses more about the significance of diet in the overall biomedical approach.

3. Detoxification (chelation or cleansing)

As you begin to decrease the allergy and inflammation through dietary control and supplementation your child can begin the process of detoxification more effectively. Detoxification is the process of cleansing toxins. Our body generates many chemicals that naturally help do this for us. The skin, intestines, liver and kidneys are the organ systems responsible for detoxification. One of the challenges with children on the spectrum is that they commonly have weakened detoxification capacity (3). Therefore, aiding their body with this process is critical.

Simple steps can be taken right now such as epsom salt baths – one to three cups in bath tub water 3 to 5 times per week has been reported to offer good results. Some parents report added benefit using sauna therapy. In home Far Infra-Red saunas are available for this purpose. There are many manufacturers of in-home saunas. I personally own a Heavenly Heat Saunas from www.heavenlysaunas.com.

Chelation therapy (aka. heavy metal detoxification therapy) is a term used to describe detoxification of heavy metal toxins such as mercury, arsenic, and lead. I employ the use of a variety of heavy metal detoxifiers such as DMPS, DMSA, and EDTA, as well as other remedies when needed such as vitamin and minerals, homeopathic and herbal medicine to assist in the detoxification process.

4. Neurological Healing and Recovery

Once your child's body has been cleared of toxins to the best of their ability they can begin the process of neurological healing and recovery.

Neurological healing involves a number of therapies known to aide the brain in injury recovery. One in particular called Hyperbaric Oxygen Therapy (HBOT) has shown great promise in aiding this process (4). This process of neurological healing is last in my list because in my experience a child will not reach their full potential unless some of the steps in the first 3 stages are implemented initially. However, this does not mean that a therapy such as HBOT could not be implemented in the early stages of biomedical intervention. In fact, HBOT has a tremendous upside with respects to improving oxygenation concentration in the brain and the reduction of neurological inflammation. This makes it beneficial in any stage of biomedical intervention.

For an excellent discussion about the benefits of HBOT therapy for autism-spectrum children see article titled *"Hyperbaric Oxygen Therapy (HBOT) for Children with Autism-Spectrum Disorders."* This can be found at Dr. Neubrander's website at www.drneubrander.com or in the Hyperbaric Oxygen Therapy section of www.AutismActionPlan.com.

NOTE: For some children these treatment steps or phases will at times overlap, with no specific dividing line between them. For example, the use of heavy metal detoxifiers with

DMSA or DMPS and the concurrent use of Hyperbaric Oxygen Treatment are many times implemented.

With regards to detoxification and/or chelation (also referred to as heavy metal detoxification) therapy, my goal is to make this a one time process, albeit for some children this process may take months to years (average time is approximately 6 months to 1 year). It is possible that some children will need to explore this avenue of treatment again to help keep their body clear of toxins.

Developing an Action Plan:

From my experience one of the unfortunate things that often occurs with parents is the "mass confusion effect" that sets in when moving down the path of biomedical intervention. People become easily confused by all the options, diets, therapies, tests, and supplements. This leads to inaction, anxiety and frustration. Ultimately, this benefits no one as you either give-up on the whole approach or never really get started with anything significant that could make a difference for your child. This has nothing to do with intelligence. It is related to the fact that the language and concepts of biomedicine are new to people.

Developing an action plan up-front will help to guide which path to take and where you should spend most of your time focusing your attention. I will give you some suggestions about how to develop your action plan. These suggestions are tried and true from my personal clinical experience and at their core level really help the majority of kids on the autistic-spectrum – and I am confident will help your child as well. All it takes is the willingness to try. Chapter 5 will give an overview of an "Action Plan" approach, while chapters 6-10 will discuss each section of the action plan more in-depth.

References:

(1) Barthelemy C, et al. Biological and clinical effects of oral magnesium and associated magnesium-vitamin B6 administration on certain disorders observed in infantile autism. *Therapie.* 1980 Sep-Oct;35(5):627-32.

(2) Neuroglial activation and neuroinflammation in the brain of patients with autism. Vargas, et al - Ann Neurol. 2005 Feb;57(2):304

(3) Alberti A, et al. Sulphation deficit in "low-functioning" autistic children: a pilot study. *Biol Psychiatry.* 1999 Aug 1;46(3):420-4.

(4) Hyperbaric oxygen therapy may improve symptoms in autistic children. Rossignol DA, Rossignol LW. Med Hypotheses 2006;67 (2):216-28.

Chapter 5

Implementing the Action Plan- "Action Steps"

Listed below are three "Action Plan" outlines which you can use as a template. The first is focused on "What You Can Do Right Now." This plan does not require any laboratory testing, nor particular input from your doctor - other than to discuss the addition or altering of your child's supplement program or medication (it is always important and recommended to discuss changes in your child's treatment program with their personal physician). No specific knowledge of biochemistry is required. All you need is access to the internet and/or a telephone.

Each plan can be supported by me with a subscription to www.AutismActionPlan.com. This biomedical resource website provides you access to in-depth information such as articles, protocols, videos, troubleshooting suggestions, and most important a member forum where you can ask questions directly to me (in private if you prefer) regarding biomedical intervention for your child.

Action plan #2 does involve some testing, but not blood testing.

Action plan #3 is more involved and requires the assistance of a physician, preferably one familiar with biomedical testing and therapies. This plan does involve blood testing. One additional therapy (discussed at the end of this chapter, and more detailed in Chapter 9) which absolutely must be considered in the beginning stages of treatment is methylcobalamin therapy (commonly called Methyl-B12 or MB-12). This therapy would generally fall under the Action Plan #2 or #3 category, but it may be implemented under Action Plan #1. However, Methyl-B12 (in the form I recommend) is a prescription item only.

(Note: downloadable prescription forms for Methyl-B12 injections and other therapies are available from www.AutismActionPlan.com. These still require a doctor's signature, but they are designed to make it easy for any willing physician to follow the directions and have it sent to a specified compounding pharmacy – listed on the prescription form).

ACTION PLAN #1 - What You Can Do Right Now!

- Begin implementing a gluten, casein and soy-free diet now! (if you are really motivated start a Specific Carbohydrate Diet or Low Oxalate Diet) – However, beginning a gluten, casein and soy-free diet is a great place to start.

- Start adding some supplements to your child's health program.

I know you all just went "phooey" (or insert another more appropriate word of choice here!). Here's another person telling me to do "The Diet" (aka. the GF/CF or gluten-free/ casein-free diet). Remember these are only suggestions, but I can tell you there is a reason almost every serious parent and/or practitioner who pursues biomedical therapies keeps telling you about this diet - because it works. That is the bottom line – it works.

Will it or will it not work for your child? Right now we do not know, and the only person you are short-changing by not implementing this diet is your child. It could turn out to be one of the most significant things you do for them. I have seen this on many occasions with patients. Parents finally implement the diet and "whammo" their kid starts getting better. I often get asked the question, "Do we need to do the diet?" My answer is "do you want to see if one of the most helpful therapies we have can work – or do you want to take the chance that it won't?" Is it a pain in the neck to do? Sometimes! Is it impossible to do? Absolutely not! Will it work for your child? I don't know – personally I would try it and see what happens.

NOTE: My Autism Action Plan website (www.AutismActionPlan.com) contains a 12 Week Action Plan outline that explains in detail how to implement the gluten and casein-free diet, as well as starting basic supplement therapy as well.

Begin administering some basic supplements

The plan right now can cause amazing changes for your child. Implementing just a change in their diet can vastly change their overall health, reduce inflammation in their digestive system and body, and improve their ability to absorb nutrients which is critical for brain development and healing.

The other thing to begin implementing is some basic supplements. These supplements provide a well rounded amount of nutrients that I have found the majority of autism-spectrum children can benefit from. The dosages are not toxic and they are *relatively* easy to get kids to take. I say relatively, because there is always going to be that one child who will throw a fit when asked (or told) to take supplements. This is one area where your determination as parent will be put to the test.

Most children need to take supplements. It is not a matter of choice. Your autistic child likely has nutritional deficiencies and imbalances that need to be corrected (1). The basic supplements I am recommending are not excessive. Remember - just because your child does not like taking supplements does not mean they know what is best for them. Most kids with Type 1 Diabetes do not like having to take their insulin injections either, but it is a matter of life and death for them. This is not to imply that your autistic child will die if they do not take supplements, but in my experience they have very little chance of improved health with respects to their autism if they do not.

In the additional resource section is an article by Lori Knowles titled "Getting Kids to Take Supplements." Read this for practical information about how to deal with a difficult child and supplements. Lori Knowles is the mother of a recovered child from autism, and she provides some practical insight from a parent who has been there with these complex issues.

There are many excellent supplement companies representing themselves to the autism community. As with any health program there are a wide variety of options. The best advice I can give is to focus your attention on building and supporting your child's overall health. You want to provide your child with the basics first. There is always time to add things later, but if you follow my recommendations your child will get the basics they need for long-term health. Remember, the basic supplements listed below are just that – the basics. I call this approach plugging holes nutritionally. What this means is these supplements can be taken by most anyone and not require an extensive laboratory assessment to determine their need. What we are looking to do is fill in the gaps nutritionally that your child may (or likely) has or is deficient in (if they are like most other ASD kids who self-limit their diet to such things as chicken nuggets, french fries and potato chips).

One supplement company I recommend is New Beginnings Nutritionals at **877-575-2467** or www.nbnus.com. The individuals at New Beginnings have a wealth of knowledge about their particular products and a unique interest in helping parents. Many of the people at New Beginnings are parents themselves of children on the autism spectrum. If you are currently not using supplements with your child, the list of supplement products below will be a good place to start. If you are currently using some supplements with your child then New Beginnings has other items which may be of interest to you.

Remember, these are only suggestions to take into consideration with respects to your child's particular needs and health condition. Please discuss all changes to your child's health program with your personal physician.

Basic Starter Program (from New Beginnings Nutritionals)

Multi Mineral & Multi Vitamin:

- Basic Nutrients Plus

Antioxidant:

- Antioxidant Formula

Liquid Mineral:

- Chelate-Mate
- Liquid Calcium
- Liquid Magnesium
- Liquid Zinc

Essential Fatty Acids with Natural Vitamin A:

- Cod Liver Oil

Probiotic:

- ProBiotic Support Formula

Alternative Approach (combining a multi mineral/vitamin/ antioxidant)

- **Syndion** – powder or capsules (this can then be combined with calcium, magnesium, cod liver oil and probiotic support formula for an overall basic supplement program.

NOTE: All of these supplements can be mixed in juice or water. Some can be easily mixed in things like pear or apple sauce.

Please see New Beginnings website (www.nbnus.com) for more specifics about dosing, timing and implementation of these supplements. There are also video explanations for most of these supplements at my supplement information website - www.AutismSupplementsCenter.com.

ACTION PLAN #2

The following is list of laboratory companies that I most commonly use in my practice.

- **BioHealth (BH)** – www.biodia.com
- **Doctors Data (DD)** – www.doctorsdata.com
- **Great Plains Laboratory (GPL)** – www.greatplainslaboratory.com

Action plan #2 includes the recommendations from Action #1 plus some basic testing (*non-blood*).

If you are in a position where you do not have the ability to order blood work (see Action Plan #3), or you would like to start some basic tests that do not require blood work then this is the plan for you. One thing to consider with respect to the development of a comprehensive program is the eventual need to do blood testing. However, this can always come later. I have seen on occasion some kids do so well with basic supplement support and dietary changes that blood work was never implemented. However, this is rare.

There can be essential information that needs to be assessed via your child's blood, i.e. mineral levels, kidney and liver function if the eventual goal is to implement heavy metal detoxification therapy, antiviral, or other detoxification therapies. In my practice, I recommend to parents to do as much testing upfront that they can afford. This way you are armed with more details of your child's specific issues and immediate needs for therapeutic intervention.

More specifics are given in Chapter 8 about diagnostic testing. However, as I have indicated the need for blood work assessment can always come later after you have started some basic intervention (see Action Plan #1). Also, another thing to consider for many young children is that there is only so much blood that can be taken at one time (based on their weight) – so this can be a limiting factor. **Testing Recommendations for Action Plan #2 (all these tests are non-blood)**

- **Comprehensive Digestive Stool Analysis w/ parasites** *(DD or GPL)*
- **Amino Acid Analysis** (DD or GPL)
- **Fecal Metals** *(DD or GPL)*
- **Hair Analysis** *(DD or GPL)*
- **Organic Acid Test** *(GPL)*
- **Porphyrin Profile** *(GPL or* Laboratoire Philippe Auguste in France – www.labbio.net).
- **Urinary Peptides** *(GPL)*

ACTION PLAN #3

Action Plan #3 involves both action plans #1 and #2. However, in addition to these is the recommendation for additional blood testing, and implementing methycobalamin (Methyl-B12) therapy.

This is my preferred path to begin. This action plan incorporates the basic supplements I recommended above, the comprehensive testing that I feel minimally should be done for most children (including the non-blood tests listed in Action Plan #2, as well as blood tests – see below), and the implementation of a highly effective therapy called Methyl-B12. Please see Chapter #10 for an in-depth discussion about Methyl-B12.

Testing Recommendations for Action Plan #3 (all these are blood tests)

NOTE: As previously stated please be aware that there is only so much blood that can be taken from one child at any one time. In my experience the tests listed below can be completed in one blood draw visit for most children. The tests labeled optional can be added on, but often will cause the amount of blood to be drawn to exceed the limit acceptable for most children. These are normally done at a later time.

- ***Packed Red Blood Cell Analysis** *(DD or GPL)*
- ***Plasma Amino Acids** *(DD or GPL)*
- ***Comprehensive Food IGG Profile** *(GPL)*
- **Other Blood Tests (most are available from standard labs: LabCorp or Quest Diagnostics:**
    - ***Comprehensive Blood Chemistry that includes electrolytes, BUN/Creatinine, and Liver Panel**
    - ***Total Cholesterol, HDL, LDL, Triglycerides (called a lipid panel)**

- *Complete Blood Count with Differential (called a CBC w/Diff)**
- *TSH, free T3, free T4** (with the addition of Anti-TPO and Anti-Thyroglobulin antibodies if autoimmune thyroiditis is a concern).
- *Serum Iron and Ferritin**
- **Total Immunoglobulins (IgG, IgM, IgA, IgE)** – Also available from Great Plains Laboratory as the Immune Deficiency Panel.
- **Rubeola (measles) titer: IgG and IgM** (Rubella levels can be added).
- **ASO (anti-streptolysin) + Anti-DNAse B** (also available from Great Plains Laboratory as the Streptococcus Panel)
- **Vitamin D as a 25(OH)D analysis** (optional)
- **ANA, Sed Rate, C-Reactive Protein** – these are markers for inflammation and autoimmune reactions (optional)
- **Viral Panel** (includes the herpes viruses – herpes 1 and 2, cytomegalovirus, epstein-barr, herpes virus 6 and varicella) – optional
- **Natural Killer Cell Analysis and activity** (optional)

- **Lymes (Borrelia burgdoferi): IgM, IgG Western Blot, Lyme IFA** (can be added if clinical suspicion is high. (*www.IgeneX.com*) – optional
- **Essential Fatty Acid Analysis** *(GPL)* – optional

NOTE: The labs tests with an asterisk (*) next to them are the ones that most commonly are ordered as an *initial* laboratory evaluation. Individual needs may vary. Labs such as **Natural Killer Cell Activity, Immunoglobulins, Streptococcus (ASO, anti-DNAseB)** and what is called a **T & B Lymphocyte Panel** are all part of the immune work-up for Neuroimmune Dysfunction as outlined by a group called Stop Calling It Autism - www.StopCallingItAutism.org.

There are a myriad of other markers that can be tested – the list is endless really, but most of the time not necessary in the beginning stages. I am presenting to you what I often use in my clinic to begin the assessment of an autistic child (or adult). What you are trying to accomplish with this initial series of tests is to establish a baseline with respects to your child's level of mineral and body chemistry function, digestive function, food sensitivities, etc. I will explain more in Chapter 7 (Diagnostic Testing) about why I recommend these tests and how they can influence your decision making with respects to biomedical intervention.

This comprehensive profile takes into account the non-blood and blood testing that is laying the immediate ground work for future therapies. Some of these therapies include anti-fungals (Nystatin, Diflucan, natural remedies such as capyrilic acid or grape seed extract), antibacterials (prescription antibiotics or natural agents), antivirals (Acyclovir, Famvir, Valtrex or natural remedies like lauricidin or Larrea Tridentata), and Transfer Factor immune support and other advanced support for heavy metal detoxification. All of these later remedies are based on what is found on the initial series of tests, and will help to determine what priority additional therapy should be implemented.

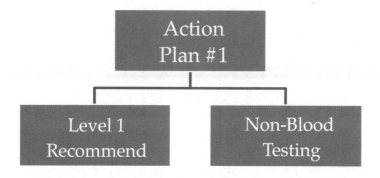

Action Plan #2 is an extension of Action Plan #1, with the addition of non-blood testing listed above.

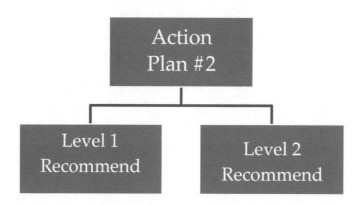

Action Plan #3 is the most comprehensive of the three because it incorporates both Action Plans 1 & 2.

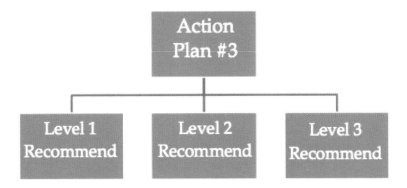

In summary, action plan #1 is the easiest of the 3. It can be viewed as a "Do It Yourself" program to start. Action Plan #3 is the most comprehensive of the three because it incorporates both action plans #1 and #2.

At the beginning of this chapter I mentioned one additional therapy I highly recommend to begin ASAP for your child called Methyl-B12 – preferably Methyl-B12 injections (nasal spray is an option, but not as good as the injections). Now, if this is the first time you are hearing about this treatment it may seem like quite a shock and raises the anxiety meter up a few notches. Do not be alarmed. This is a normal response for most parents until they realize how easy and fantastic this treatment can be. For a more detailed discussion about Methyl-B12 therapy please see Chapter 9.

For now, suffice it to say that if someone came into my office and told me "Doctor Woeller, we are going to take everything away from you that you use to treat autistic kids, except a few things - what would you keep?" Hands down I would keep Methyl-B12 injections (as well as therapy called Respen-A – see Chapter 10 for this important treatment too). The Methyl-B12 treatment is <u>that</u> important. Kind of peaked your interest didn't I? Well, before you immediately flip to Chapter 9 (which you absolutely need to read) take a look at the graph below. We can now take our Action Plans 1, 2, 3 and incorporate Methyl-B12 into the mix.

As you can see this opens up a number of options in the early stages of a biomedical program for your child. This is commonly a place that I start with in my practice. One of the most important things to keep in mind about adding Methyl-B12 therapy to your child's treatment program, whether it is done right now or sometime later is that it is done as a *stand alone* treatment for at least 6 weeks with no other supplements, dietary changes, or medications added at that same time (unless of course there is an emergency such as an accident or infection requiring prescription medication). This does not mean you would stop other treatment you are currently doing. You just do not want to add anything "new" to your child's program during the first 6 weeks of the Methyl-B12 protocol. The reason is simple. You want to see if your child is a Methyl-B12 responder. This has been such an important therapy that you want to make sure you get a clear picture of its benefits right from the beginning.

A common scenario in my practice is as follows. This is only an example and at times is altered based on an individual child's needs.

Scenario #1: No Supplements, No Testing, Have Not Implemented Special Diet:

- Begin Methyl-B12 ASAP
- Start test collections ASAP
- Implement GF/CF diet and supplements after first 6 weeks of Methyl-B12

Scenario #2: Currently on Supplements, No Testing, Have Not Implemented Special Diet:

- Stay on current supplements
- Begin Methyl-B12 ASAP
- Start test collections ASAP
- Implement diet and supplement changes (if indicated) after first 6 weeks of Methyl-B12.

Scenario #3: Currently on Special Diet, i.e. GF/CF and Supplements, No Testing:

- Begin Methyl-B12 ASAP
- Start test collections ASAP
- Implement diet (switch to SCD or LOD) and supplement changes (if indicated) after first 6 weeks of Methyl-B12.

In some circumstances, parents will like to wait on starting Methyl-B12, or need a little more time to research - this is okay. I am always in favor of parents being comfortable with the therapies they are giving. The best place to get more specific information about how to implement this therapy is on my biomedical subscription website at www.AutismActionPlan.com. Additional information can be accessed from Dr. Neubrander's website (father of Methyl-B12 therapy for autism) at www.drneubrander.com.

If you decide to wait on Methyl-B12 therapy then the implementation of Action Plans #1, #2, and #3 are still available to you. My recommendation is that if you have not implemented a specific diet, such as GF/CF or SCD (see Chapter 8 for more details) and/or basic supplements - get going now! There is nothing wrong with this basic approach.

The most important thing to remember with respect to biomedical intervention is – *to do something*. Even little changes can make a big difference. Special diets, supplements, and testing are all part of the program overtime. The more you do simultaneously over time, the better chance you have at helping your child improve.

References:

(1)- Adams JB, Holloway C. Pilot study of a moderate dose multivitamin/mineral supplement for children with autistic spectrum disorder. *J Altern Complement Med.* 2004 Dec;10(6):1033-9.

Chapter 6
Information is Power

Getting Informed

This action step is absolutely critical if you are going to be successful in helping your child on the biomedical path. You have to be informed, and you have to take it upon yourself to become educated about biomedical intervention for autism. I cannot say it any other way, but those who are unwilling to get in the game and begin the process of self-education will forever stand on the sidelines and never see much success with their children using biomedical therapies.

There is no biomedical autism doctor or other health practitioner that can do it all for you. You have to research and be willing to try new things with your child. There is a lot of support regarding biomedical information about therapies, testing, etc., available through support group organizations, such as TACA (www.tacanow.org), other online websites and chat groups. See Yahoo! Groups for a variety of topics – for example, topics on chelation therapy, low oxalate and specific carbohydrate diet, Methyl-B12 and more. There are also biomedical conferences – Autism Research Institute, Great Plains, National Autism Association and Autism One. However, you will not find much available through mainstream press or traditional physician journals.

Remember that you are your child's best advocate. No one else can do it for you. You can do it. You have it in you. You

just have to open your mind to the possibilities and be willing to try new things. There is plenty of assistance available in the autism community - just reach out and someone will be willing to help. Again, I am available as well through my
subscription biomedical website at
www.AutismActionPlan.com.

This chapter is an outline of the various books, DVDs, biomedical conferences, and support organizations that I feel are critical for your education process. Becoming familiar with a broad spectrum of viewpoints and information will better allow you to help your child.

Reference Books:

There are many fine books to choose from regarding biomedical therapies:

- **"Biological Treatments for Autism and PDD"** by William Shaw, Ph.D. – can be ordered online at www.greatplainslaboratory.com. **This is a high priority book and was one of the first books I read to better understand what biomedical therapies have to offer the autism community.**

- **"Unraveling the Mystery of Autism and Pervasive Developmental Disorder"** by Karyn Seroussi. A very nice introduction to the principles of why biomedicine can be helpful. Specifically highlights the benefits of the gluten and casein-free diet.

- **"Autism: Effective Biomedical Treatments"** by Jon Pangborn, Ph.D. and Sidney MacDonald Baker, M.D. This is a very comprehensive overview of the science behind the biomedical options that are available for treatment. This is a *must* book to have in your library. It is a useful and quick resource manual.

- **"Children with Starving Brains: A Medical Treatment Guide for Autism-Spectrum Disorders" by Jacquelyn McCandless, M.D.** This book is a wealth of information. Well written and easy to understand.

- **TACA's Autism Journey Guide** (www.tacanow.org) – TACA is the premier parent support group organization. This book is an excellent guide to various aspects of autism treatment – not just biomedical, but other avenues as well, including speech and behavioral therapy.

- **"The Puzzle of Autism" by Amy Yasko, Ph. D** – Dr. Amy Yasko has contributed much to the field of biomedicine for autism. Her work takes some time to integrate and understand, but it will be well worth the effort.

NOTE: There are many other books in print, but those listed above are the ones that I am most familiar with and have used throughout the years to expand my knowledge.

Online Resources:

There are literally hundreds of online resources that discuss autism and the variety of treatments available. Listed below are a few you should consider:

- **Autism Action Plan** – www.AutismActionPlan.com – tremendous resource of practical biomedical information and access to me (Dr. Woeller) through the Parent Forum. This website also has protocols, articles, informational audio recordings, and much more.

- **Autism Recovery Treatment** www.autismrecoverytreatment – FREE video and article blog site produced by me (Dr. Woeller) to support ongoing education information for autism.

- **Autism Research Institute** www.autismresearchinstitute.com - Must read articles on yeast/candida, vitamin therapy, heavy metal toxicity, chelation therapy, Gluten/Casein-Free Diet. **Good place to start regarding articles concerning the DAN! (Defeat Autism Now!) organization.**

- **Great Plains Laboratory** www.greatplainslaboratory.com – Excellent resource for the testing offered by Great Plains – plus special topics by Dr. Bill Shaw, including monthly web conferences. **I perform a FREE monthly web presentation on biomedical topics through Great**

Plains. Go to their website and sign up for their FREE monthly webinar service.

- **Stop Calling It Autism** www.stopcallingitautism.org - non-profit organization dedicating to dispelling the myth autism is a neurodevelopmental disorder. There primary focus is to bring attention that for many with autism they have an neuro-immune dysfunction.

- **TACA** *(Talk About Curing Autism)* www.tacanow.org – this website's information is critical for any parent wishing to access additional resources regarding biomedical therapies, as well as other important information regarding the care, education, and special needs of an autism-spectrum child.

Biomedical Conferences and Seminars:

These are extremely useful to help you better understand that the therapies, tests, and dietary recommendations we make are rooted in science and research. We are not talking about "far out stuff" here! Everything we do has a specific purpose. Whether it is to correct a nutritional deficiency or support a defective biochemical pathway, it all has meaning.

Conferences that support the biomedical approach are a great place to find the latest research in biomedical treatment for autism. This does not mean that other conferences about autism are not worthwhile - they are.

However, the majority of parents who are dealing with autism in their lives are not even aware of the biomedical options available for their children. What a shame!

- **Autism Research Institute Conferences -** Conferences dedicated to biomedical treatment and research for autism and autism-spectrum disorders. This is both a physician and parent oriented seminar. Contact the Autism Research Institute at www.autismresearchinstitute.com. Conferences are held twice yearly on both the east and west of the U.S.

- **Great Plains Laboratory Biomedical Conferences –** Contact Great Plains Laboratory at www.greatplainslaboratory.com for upcoming conferences.

- **USAAA (United States Autism & Asperger's Association)** www.usaaa.org - conference that incorporates biomedical and non-biomedical therapy.

- **Autism One** - conference that incorporates traditional biomedical therapy as well as more holistic approaches such as herbs, and homeopathy, www.autismone.org

Join and Attend Parent Support Groups:

These are an invaluable service for parents. Most support groups hold monthly meetings and provide a tremendous amount of information regarding therapy resources, educational services, literature, etc. The most recognized support group network is TACA (Talk About Curing Autism). Being familiar with TACA and using their services is essential for any parent new to the biomedical approach - even if you live outside the Southern California area of the United States (where TACA is headquartered):

- **Talk About Curing Autism (TACA)**
  www.tacanow.org

I am a huge proponent of parent education. You have to be your own independent researcher – there is too much at stake. You do not have to become an expert in every subject, but in looking back on the kids who have done very well with biomedical therapies, particularly those who have lost their diagnosis or became indistinguishable from their peers it was because of their parents who stayed on top of the information and implemented the therapies. The important thing is to begin the process. Be patient with yourself and allow for your education to grow over time. Self-education is powerful and necessary, but it is also a process.

Chapter 7
Diagnostic Testing Options

In this chapter I will discuss more in depth the basic (or introductory) testing I commonly recommend. Much of this testing is recommended to do up-front to get a comprehensive overview of your child's health status. As with anything in medicine, diagnostic testing is a dynamic science that is constantly advancing in its ability to evaluate various aspects of our body's reactions to environmental stressors, as well as internal metabolic changes. The testing that I describe in this chapter is a list of the most commonly utilized tests in my practice. This chapter is meant to be used as a guide to help you get started in evaluating your child. If you are working with your personal physician, they can contact each laboratory individually and set up accounts for test kit ordering.

Everyone Must Be Involved

It is imperative that everyone involved in your child's health care understand that the evaluation and treatment for children with autism is a process and not an event. Please understand that this process takes time and the length of time is different for every child. There are no magic bullets.

The Importance of Testing

Comprehensive analysis and sophisticated treatment protocols are essential to address the varied medical issues of your child. This section will describe 3 different "pathways" or testing options I have developed. Each option will provide comprehensive analysis of your child's body systems from metabolic function, toxicity from heavy metals, yeast assessment and more. Each option or pathway has been developed to allow for immediate implementation of therapies such as anti-fungal treatment, vitamin and mineral support, Methyl-B12 treatment, Respen-A, general and heavy metal detoxification therapy (aka. chelation). The main difference between the various options is the comprehensiveness of testing data that is collected and the price for each option (pricing is approximate as prices for labs do change with time). Obviously, the more testing that is performed the better assessment you can make.

Unfortunately, many of the tests and therapies that are recommended may not be covered by your insurance (please see section below under "Cost and Pricing"). **This does not mean that the tests are not insurance reimbursable.** I encourage everyone to try and submit to their insurance carrier. Each lab is different so you will need to check with them and inquire about their policy for insurance billing. Many people are successful in getting reimbursement. However, it depends entirely on your individual insurance plan. Also, many of the test panels are specialized diagnostics and may not available through your standard HMO or PPO medical services.

Listed below is a list of very important points with regards to my laboratory testing procedure:

- The test panels I generally use in my practice are available from three major laboratory companies:

BioHealth, Doctor's Data, and Great Plains Laboratory. Other labs such as IgeneX (Lyme testing), Great Smokies Diagnostics, Neuroimmunology, SpectraCell Laboratories and/or Dr. Yasko (genetic profiling) are also used as needed.

- For a variety of standard blood tests such as liver and kidney function, cholesterol, thyroid, electrolyte (sodium, potassium) levels, etc., are available from standard reference labs such as Lab Corp and Quest Diagnostics. Your local hospital or HMO/PPO laboratories may be able to perform some of these tests as well. Also, these labs are generally used to assist in the collection of blood samples for the specialized blood test kits from the aforementioned laboratory companies: BioHealth, Doctor's Data, Great Plains Laboratory, and others.

IMPORTANT NOTE:

In my practice, the specialized laboratory tests kits we provide can be sent to your home for in-home collection (hair, urine, and stool) or taken to a local blood draw station such as a hospital or clinic. If your pediatrician or family physician has blood draw services in their office, they can help you with this as well. Once the test kit samples are collected you will be responsible for mailing them to the respective labs (in some cases the blood draw facility will do this for you). Detailed instructions are found within each lab test kit about collection and mailing.

My advice is to read the instructions for each test kit – *carefully and thoroughly.* This is critically important to make sure test collections are done correctly. Many people are accustomed to their regular physician's office handling all testing. However, because the laboratory tests that I recommend are specialized, it requires your involvement in making sure collecting, handling and shipping requirements are done correctly.

NOTE: In the www.AutismActionPlan.com website under the Lab Ordering section (which provides access to the Organic Acid Test and Comprehensive Digestive Stool Analysis from Great Plains Laboratory) there are sample videos of how to do test collection.

Cost of Tests

The process of biomedical assessment and treatment for children on the autism-spectrum can be time consuming and financially challenging. It is important that you as a parent or caregiver be informed upfront what financial commitments you will be facing when deciding what diagnostic tests to perform for your child. It is impossible for me or anyone else to give exact figures regarding costs for all testing, supplements, medications and consults as each child is unique and will require different therapy. However, I have provided an estimation of costs to consider when evaluating diagnostic testing. It is important to recognize that some insurance companies do reimburse for much of the testing and consult fees that are required for your child. Medications and supplements vary, and depend upon your specific insurance carrier, but it is not unreasonable to assume that many insurance plans (particularly PPO's) will reimburse for at least 50% of your child's medical costs.

Each testing option or pathway has an approximate cost attached to it. **This price is for the cost of the tests** *ONLY.* **It does not include costs for consult fees for test interpretation and review, supplements and medications.** These additional costs are variable depending upon the extent of interventions your child needs. Of course, you as a parent or caregiver make the decision regarding what therapies you want to apply for your child, and how much you can afford.

Test Panel Options

Please note that when considering test panels it is a good idea to get as much information upfront as possible. One major reason is to quickly determine what your child's health priorities are. The more information you have, the quicker you can begin implementing specific targeted therapies. This saves time and money and allows for you to utilize the majority of your financial resources on therapy. Also, for most individuals, the testing options listed below are only needed once.

There will always be some tests that need to be looked at again, but this is on an individual basis and for most individuals, they are not re-doing extensive tests panels over and over.

There are four different options. Test panels #1-3 all require blood. Test panel #4 is stool, hair and urine only. Remember that whichever panel you choose - significant information can be ascertained and the ability to implement important therapies such as Methyl-B12 therapy, Respen-A, and basic vitamin/mineral supplements is always available prior to doing any testing.

CRITICAL POINT - *These test panel recommendations can always be modified as needed to meet your child's specific needs and your financial situation.*

OPTION #1 – Advanced Comprehensive (blood testing required)

This pathway is the obvious preferred pathway for the most in-depth and comprehensive testing of all panels discussed. It provides a detailed analysis of your child's digestive function, blood chemistry, food sensitivity and yeast status. It incorporates specialized tests with regards to heavy metal toxicity and exposure, mineral and amino acid status, viruses, and immune system function. This profile aids in decision making regarding which therapies will best suit your child. With this analysis you can prioritize the need for detoxification support therapies such as DMPS, DMSA, EDTA, anti-fungals concerning non-systemic medication (Nystatin) versus systemic (Diflucan), and antibacterial and/or parasitic treatment and Borrelia (Lymes). With this analysis you can better differentiate the need for neurochemical support, streptococcal bacteria intervention and the potential benefit of therapies such as antiviral medication and/or Intravenous Immunoglobulin Therapy (IVIG):

- **Viral Titers, including Natural Killer Cell Analysis** *(blood) – available from most laboratories such as LabCorp and Quest Diagnostics (includes herpes 1 and 2, Cytomegalovirus, Epstein-Barr, HHV6 , Measles and*

Varicella IgG, IgM antibodies. Also, adding a Sublymphocyte and Natural Killer Cell analysis is desirable) – evaluates herpes viruses, Natural Killer Cells and chicken pox and measles antibodies.

- **Amino Acid Analysis** *(blood)* – evaluates for circulating levels of amino acids (building blocks of proteins), abnormalities, and deficiencies.
- **Comprehensive Blood Chemistry** *(blood)*:
  - Electrolytes, i.e. sodium, potassium, kidney function (BUN, creatinine) and liver enzymes (AST, ALT).
  - Complete Blood Count with Differential, i.e. lymphocytes, monocytes.
  - Total Cholesterol, LDL, HDL, triglycerides
  - Thyroid Evaluation – TSH (thyroid stimulating hormone), free T3, free T4 anti-TPO and anti-thyroglobulin (if concerned about autoimmune thyroid condition)
  - Serum Iron and Ferritin
  - Vitamin D as a 25 (OH) D analysis
  - C-Reactive Protein
  - Serum Homocysteine
  - ASO (anti-streptolysin) and Anti-DNAse B (especially if history of Obsessive-Compulsive Disorder and/or Tics) or chronic infections.

NOTE: These test markers can be performed by most reference labs such as LabCorp, Quest, and others. These can all be prescribed by your personal physician. The remaining tests listed are considered more specialized.

- **Comprehensive Digestive Stool Analysis w/parasite** *(stool)* – stool test that evaluates for the presence of yeast, bacteria, parasites and markers for intestinal inflammation and digestion.

- **Comprehensive Food IgG** *(blood)* – evaluates sensitivity to over 90 different foods.
- **Copper/Zinc Profile (blood)** – evaluates for the level of copper, zinc and ceruloplasmin indicating potential imbalances in copper metabolism.
- **Fecal Metals** *(stool)* – stool analysis to determine environmental exposures of heavy metals.
- **Hair Analysis** *(hair)* – shows imbalances of minerals that indicates the presence of heavy metals.
- **Immune Deficiency Panel (blood)** – evaluates for total antibody (IgG, IgM, IgA, IgE) production and potential for deficiencies.
- **Organic Acid Test** *(urine)* – evaluates for yeast and bacterial toxins, metabolic imbalances.
- **Porphyrin Profile** *(urine)* – evaluates for porphyrin metabolism which is essential for hemoglobin production (carries oxygen). Porphyrins are a significant marker for heavy metal toxicity.
- **Red Blood Cell Mineral Assessment** *(blood)* – evaluates mineral levels. Important for any detoxification program.
- **Urinary Peptide** *(urine)* – evaluates for peptides (morphine-like chemicals) of gluten and casein.

Approximate Test Panel Price = $3000 to $3500

Add-On Testing:

- **Initial Lyme IgG, IgM Western Blot and Lyme IFA** *(blood)* – evaluates for immune markers for the presence of Lyme (Borrelia) spirochete which is present

in some kids with autism. The Borrelia bacteria can be passed during pregnancy.
- **Essential Fatty Analysis** *(blood)* – evaluates for deficiencies and imbalances in essential fatty acids.
- **Folate Receptor Antibodies (blood)**

OPTION #2 – Comprehensive *(blood testing required)*

This pathway is another preferred pathway regarding in-depth and comprehensive testing. It is an excellent place to start particularly if you prefer to analyze your child's food sensitivity prior to implementing a gluten, casein and soy-free diet. It provides a detailed analysis of your child's digestive function, blood chemistry, food sensitivity and yeast status. It incorporates specialized tests with regards to heavy metal exposure, mineral and amino acid status, and viruses. This profile aids in the decision making regarding which therapies will best suit your child. With this analysis you can prioritize the need for mineral and amino acid support, anti-fungals concerning non-systemic medication (Nystatin) versus systemic (Diflucan), and antibacterial and/or parasitic treatment. With this analysis you are also able to better differentiate the potential benefits of therapies such as antiviral medication.

- **Amino Acid Analysis** *(blood)* – evaluates for circulating levels of amino acids (building blocks of proteins), abnormalities, and deficiencies.
- **Comprehensive Blood Chemistry** *(blood)*:
  - Electrolytes, i.e. sodium, potassium, kidney function (BUN, creatinine) and liver enzymes (AST, ALT).

- Complete Blood Count with Differential, i.e. lymphocytes, monocytes.
- Total Cholesterol, LDL, HDL, triglycerides
- Thyroid Evaluation – TSH (thyroid stimulating hormone), free T3, free T4 anti-TPO and anti-thyroglobulin (if concerned about autoimmune thyroid condition)
- Serum Iron and Serum Ferritin
- Vitamin D as a 25 (OH) D analysis
- C-Reactive Protein
- Serum Homocysteine
- Rubeola (measles) IgG
- ASO (anti-streptolysin) and Anti-DNAse B (especially if there is a history of Obsessive-Compulsive Disorder, Tics or chronic infections).

NOTE: These test markers can be performed by most reference labs such as LabCorp, Quest, and others. These can all be prescribed by your personal physician. The remaining labs listed are considered more specialized laboratory tests.

- **Comprehensive Digestive Stool Analysis w/parasite** *(stool)* – stool test that evaluates for the presence of yeast, bacteria, parasites and markers for intestinal inflammation and digestion.
- **Comprehensive Food IgG** *(blood)* – evaluates sensitivity to over 90 different foods.
- **Copper/Zinc Profile (blood)** – evaluates for the level of copper, zinc and ceruloplasmin indicating potential imbalances in copper metabolism.

- **Fecal Metals** *(stool)* – stool analysis to determine environmental exposures to heavy metals.
- **Hair Analysis** *(hair)* – shows imbalances of minerals that indicates the presence of heavy metals.
- **Immune Deficiency Panel (blood)** – evaluates for total antibody (IgG, IgM, IgA, IgE) production and potential for deficiencies.
- **Organic Acid Test** *(urine)* – evaluates for yeast and bacterial toxins, metabolic imbalances.
- **Porphyrin Profile** *(urine)* – evaluates for porphyrin metabolism which is essential for hemoglobin production (carries oxygen). Porphyrins are a significant marker for heavy metal toxicity.
- **Red Blood Cell Mineral Assessment** *(blood)* – evaluates mineral levels. Important for any detoxification program.
- **Urinary Peptide** *(urine)* – evaluates for peptides (morphine-like chemicals) of gluten and casein.
- **Viral Titers, including Natural Killer Cell Analysis** *(blood)* – *available from most laboratories such as LabCorp (includes herpes 1 and 2, Cytomegalovirus, Epstein-Barr, HHV6 , Measles and Varicella IgG, IgM antibodies. Also, adding a Sublymphocyte and Natural Killer Cell analysis is desirable)* – evaluates herpes viruses, Natural Killer Cells and chicken pox and measles antibodies .

Approximate Test Panel Price = $2200 to $2700

Add-On Testing:

- **Initial Lyme IgG, IgM Western Blot and Lyme IFA** *(blood)* – evaluates for immune markers for the presence of Lyme (borrelia) spirochete which is present in some kids with autism. The Borrelia bacteria can be passed during pregnancy.
- **Essential Fatty Analysis** *(blood)* – evaluates for deficiencies and imbalances in essential fatty acids.
- **Cerebral Folate Antibodies (blood)**

OPTION #3 – Basic *(blood testing required)*

This pathway is a fine place to start, particularly if you do not need to be convinced of the benefits of the gluten, casein, and soy-free diet, or have already implemented specialized diets. This panel provides detailed analysis of your child's digestive function, blood chemistry, food sensitivity, and yeast status. It aids in the decision making regarding which therapies will best suit your child. This profile does not allow for in-depth analysis of viral or immune status. Testing regarding heavy metal toxicity is assessed by the porphyrin profile. Heavy metal detoxification therapy <u>may</u> still be implemented based on the laboratory results from this panel of tests.

- **Amino Acid Analysis** *(blood)* – evaluates for circulating levels of amino acids (building blocks of proteins), abnormalities, and deficiencies.
- **Comprehensive Blood Chemistry** *(blood)*.

- Electrolytes, i.e. sodium, potassium, kidney function (BUN, creatinine) and liver enzymes (AST, ALT).
- Complete Blood Count with Differential, i.e. lymphocytes, monocytes.
- Total Cholesterol, LDL, HDL, triglycerides
- Thyroid Evaluation – TSH (thyroid stimulating hormone), free T3, free T4 anti-TPO and anti-thyroglobulin (if concerned about autoimmune thyroid condition)
- Serum Iron and Ferritin
- Vitamin D as a 25 (OH) D analysis
- C-Reactive Protein
- Serum Homocysteine
- Rubeola (measles) IgG
- ASO (anti-streptolysin) and Anti-DNAse B (especially if there is a history of Obsessive-Compulsive Disorder, Tics or chronic infections).

NOTE: These test markers can be performed by most reference labs such as LabCorp, Quest, and others. They can all be prescribed by your personal physician. The remaining tests listed are considered more specialized.

- **Comprehensive Digestive Stool Analysis w/parasite (stool)** – stool test that evaluates for the presence of yeast, bacteria, parasites and markers for intestinal inflammation and digestion.
- **Copper/Zinc Profile (blood)** – evaluates for the level of copper, zinc and ceruloplasmin indicating potential imbalances in copper metabolism.

- **Fecal Metals** *(stool)* – stool analysis to determine environmental exposures of heavy metals.
- **Hair Analysis** *(hair)* – shows imbalances of minerals that indicates the presence of heavy metals.
- **Organic Acid Test** *(urine)* – evaluates for yeast and bacterial toxins, metabolic imbalances.
- **Porphyrin Profile** *(urine)* – evaluates for porphyrin metabolism which is essential for hemoglobin production (carries oxygen). Porphyrins are a significant marker for heavy metal toxicity.
- **Red Blood Cell Mineral Assessment** *(blood)* – evaluates mineral levels. Important for any detoxification program.

Add-On Testing:

- **Initial Lyme IgG, IgM Western Blot and Lyme IFA** *(blood)* – evaluates for immune markers for the presence of Lyme (borrelia) spirochete. The Borrelia bacteria can be passed during pregnancy.
- **Essential Fatty Analysis** *(blood)* – evaluates for deficiencies and imbalances in essential fatty acids.
- **Cerebral Folate Receptor Antibodies**

Approximate Test Panel Price = $1500 to 1800

OPTION #4 – Very Basic _(NO BLOOD testing required)_

This pathway is a fine place as well to start, particularly if you do not need convincing regarding the benefits of the gluten, casein, and soy-free diet, or have already implemented specialized diets for your child. This is also an easy place to start without performing blood tests. You can still implement therapy such as Methyl-B12, Respen-A, and dietary supplements. This panel provides detailed analysis of your child's digestive function and yeast status. This panel is an option I often use in my practice, particularly for children who are extremely stressed by blood work and/or families on a tight budget.

This profile aids in the decision making regarding which therapies will best suit your child. This profile does not allow for an in-depth analysis of viral or immune status. Heavy metal toxicity is assessed by the porphyrin profile, but implementing intravenous heavy metal detoxification therapy using standard dosing of DMPS or EDTA cannot be started at this point (in my opinion) as it always requires blood testing for mineral, kidney and liver function status beforehand. It is possible to use low dose DMSA dosing (0.625 to 1.25mg/kg) with this testing approach under the supervision of a qualified physician.

- **Comprehensive Digestive Stool Analysis w/parasite _(stool)_** – stool test that evaluates for the presence of yeast, bacteria, parasites and markers for intestinal inflammation and digestion.

- **Fecal Metals** *(stool)* – stool analysis to determine environmental exposures of heavy metals.
- **Hair Analysis** *(hair)* – shows imbalances of minerals that indicates presence of heavy metals.
- **Organic Acid Test** *(urine)* – evaluates for yeast and bacterial toxins, metabolic imbalances.
- **Porphyrin Profile** *(urine)* – evaluates for porphyrin metabolism which is essential for hemoglobin production (carries oxygen). Porphyrins are a significant marker for heavy metal toxicity.

Approximate Test Panel Price = $1000 to 1200

IMPORTANT NOTE:

All of these test panels can be modified based on your child's needs and your financial situation. All test kits are available individually.

However, it is important to remember that certain tests are necessary in order to implement more advanced therapies such as heavy metal detoxification (DMSA, DMPS), prescription anti-fungals (anti-yeast), or specialized amino acids blends. As I have stated before it is possible to implement certain therapies like dietary changes including the gluten/casein/soy-free diet, the Specific Carbohydrate Diet (SCD), or the low-oxalate diet (LOD), Methyl-B12 therapy, Respen-A and basic supplements without doing any initial testing. However, in order to move into more advanced programs such as heavy metal detoxification (chelation therapy) each child will need to have blood testing done (blood chemistry profile including liver and kidney function, as well as mineral status, i.e. Red Blood Cell

Analysis), particularly if this therapy is being done intravenously.

Depending on your child's weight and age, tests requiring blood may not all be able to be done at one time. The reasoning is that only so much blood can be safely taken from a child at any one time.

Testing Profile - Dr. Amy Yasko Genetic Analysis

For those of you who are new to biomedicine for autism the scope of information available can at first be overwhelming - testing, treatments, supplements, and diet. Also, like anything in medicine, information changes all the time. New things are discovered, and what was thought to work yesterday is no longer applicable today. This is just the way it is in medicine – there are always changes.

Genetic profiling is an area of medicine that is gaining popularity and has the potential for wide sweeping applications regarding a host of health conditions such as predicting cardiovascular disease or susceptibility to cancer. In the biomedical field of autism, genetics and their influence over biochemical function in the child's body is well accepted. What is challenging is how to best evaluate and apply treatment based on specific test results.

One biomedical approach that can be useful is from the work of Dr. Amy Yasko. Her depth of knowledge regarding the intricacies and patterns of nutritional imbalances, detoxification issues, viral and heavy metal toxicities is extensive. In this book I am not going to go in depth into Dr. Yasko's work, but for more information you can reference her website at www.holistichealth.com. Her literature is detailed and will take some time to understand, but it is worth investigating – particularly if your child is not making good progress with standard biomedical therapies.

Dr. Yasko has a test panel that looks at various biochemical genetic markers that can indicate problem areas for your child.

These problem areas can help fine tune nutritional programs pinpointing certain supplements that could work well for your child, and which may cause a problem. In my experience many parents have implemented the above listed tests I have just discussed, and then at some point ordered Dr. Yasko's panel. However, there is no problem in doing her panel in the beginning as well.

Dr. Yasko Genetic Profile:

- **Yasko Genetic Profile** – for more information about the "Yasko Protocol" access her information at www.holistichealth.com.

Final Comment:

Try not to be overwhelmed with all the various options available regarding testing. At first glance, some people think they have to have thousands of dollars to be able to start biomedical therapies. This is not true. As stated in Chapter #6, you can easily implement a phase #1 program of dietary changes, basic supplements, and even Methyl-B12 therapy (injections via a prescription by your physician) without doing any testing in the beginning.

However, diagnostic testing is an important part of biomedical intervention for most children. Often, the decision between one option and the next comes down to finances. Ultimately, the most important part of a biomedical approach is to start doing something, anything – diet, supplements, etc., but just start.

If you are only able to afford one test in the beginning, I would recommend the Organic Acid Test (OAT) from Great Plains Laboratory. If you can afford two tests, then I would recommend the OAT and Comprehensive Stool Analysis (Great Plains Laboratory). If more tests are available to you financially – great! This gives you more options.

DIAGNOSTIC TESTS – Overview of the tests that I recommend in my various testing options.

The following is a brief discussion of the various tests and their corresponding laboratories. This is not a complete list of all tests that are available regarding biomedical assessment, but are the most commonly ordered labs for autism-spectrum children in my clinic.

- BioHealth (BH) – www.biodia.com
- Doctors Data (DD) – www.doctorsdata.com
- Great Plains Laboratory (GPL) – www.greatplainslaboratory.com

URINE

☐ **Organic Acid Test (GPL)** - This test determines biochemical and metabolic imbalances, and the presence of toxins released from certain infectious bacteria and candida. The overgrowth of these organisms can cause significant neurological problems in susceptible individuals.

☐ **Porphyrin Profile (GPL or Laboratoire Philippe Auguste in France** – www.labbio.net**)** evaluates for porphyrin metabolism which is essential for hemoglobin production (carries oxygen). Porphyrins are a significant marker for heavy metal toxicity.

☐ **Urinary Peptide (GPL)** – This test evaluates abnormal and normal levels of gliadorphin (gluten peptides) and casomorphin (casein peptides) that are commonly elevated in autistic-spectrum individuals. Research has shown these chemicals have an adverse drug-like effect on the brain similar to opiate medications such as morphine.

☐ **Urine Heavy Metal Analysis (DD, GPL)** - Urine testing to determine if your child's body has increased storage and tissue burden from heavy metals (mercury, aluminum, nickel, cadmium, etc.). This test is generally part of my heavy metal detoxification program. However, it can be performed as a baseline test using a bolus dose of DMSA or DMPS to evaluate the overall load of heavy metals.

☐ **Amino Acid Analysis (DD, GPL)** - This test is used to evaluate excess or deficiency of amino acids. Amino acids are key nutrients for cellular function, enzyme pathways, and neurochemical production. This test is generally done after improving digestive function and nutritional/dietary status.

STOOL

☐ **Gastrointestinal Pathogen Screen** (BH) – Gastrointestinal infections pose an ever increasing threat to the U.S. population. Due to globalization and international travel, parasitic infections are commonly found in all countries. This problem is especially insidious due to the fact that the absence of GI symptoms does not rule out the presence of these potentially life-threatening infectious organisms. This GI Pathogen screen determines the existence of abnormal bacteria, yeast, fungus, and parasites. Eradication of these infections is vital in order to return a patient to full health.

☐ **H. Pylori Stool Antigen (BH)** – evaluates for the presence of helicobacter pylori bacteria in the intestinal tract. A positive marker indicates an active infection.

☐ **Comprehensive Digestive Stool Analysis (DD, GPL)** – Evaluates for yeast, bacteria, parasites and markers of digestion, absorption, and inflammation.

☐ **Fecal Metals (DD, GPL)** – Stool analysis that evaluates the level of heavy metals, i.e. lead, arsenic, mercury in the stool.

BLOOD

☐ **Comprehensive Blood Chemistry (BH, Labcorp, Quest, Diagnostics)** - This comprehensive blood chemistry profile includes a complete blood count, liver enzymes, kidney function, lipid (blood fats), thyroid, and anemia profiles.

☐ **90 Food Antigen Test (GPL)** – This is a comprehensive food sensitivity test using IgG antibodies to 90 different foods.

☐ **Red Blood Cell Mineral Analysis** **(DD, GPL)** – This test assesses mineral levels. It is necessary to determine the levels of these nutrients in your child's body for heavy metal chelation. This test is commonly used when performing chelation (heavy metal detoxification) therapy with DMSA or DMPS.

☐ **Streptococcus Panel** **(GPL, Labcorp, Quest Diagnostics)** – evaluates markers of ASO and anti-DNAse B. Both are indicators of streptococcal infection (a potential contributor to obsessive-compulsive disorder).

HAIR

☐ **Hair Analysis** **(DD, GPL)** – hair analysis is a screening test for heavy metal exposure. It is a non-invasive and inexpensive way of assessing potential heavy metal toxicity and mineral status for selenium, copper and lithium.

Chapter 8
Healthy Diet is Essential
What Your Child Eats Really Does Make a Difference

As unpopular as this topic is, dietary restrictions really can make a big difference in your child's health - <u>many times dramatically!</u> Gluten (from wheat) and casein (from dairy) are two of the most common food offenders for autism-spectrum individuals (1). Soy is often times a problem as well. The gluten/casein-free diet has been used for many years with good success - many times great success. I see so many children (at least 65-70%) that have shown improvement with cognitive changes (better attention, ability to focus, language) and physical health (better digestive function, less illnesses such as colds, ear infections) that I feel a gluten, casein, and soy-free diet (GF/CF and SF) is absolutely warranted.

It Isn't Just About Gluten & Casein-free Cookies, Cakes & Sweet Treats

Food, in general, is important to evaluate with regards to overall health. The majority of autism-spectrum children are dealing with high toxin levels in their bodies which they are not able to eliminate effectively (2). A healthy diet is one way to increase essential nutrients such as vitamins, minerals, amino acids, essential fats and antioxidants that go a long way in supporting health. The gluten and casein-free diet is a good place to a start. However, I have seen parents implement this diet (with fairly good success), but never really improve the quality of food they are feeding their children.

When I talk about implementing a GF/CF diet, it's not just about gluten and casein-free cookies, cakes and sweet treats. Beyond the GF/CF diet, you should be incorporating as much organic fruits, vegetables and meats (if not vegetarian) as possible. This is critical, because these foods will contain the highest content of essential nutrients and are without the harmful addition of hormones, antibiotics, artificial coloring, flavorings and excess sugar that so many refined and processed foods contain. The removal of toxic food such as fast-food (junk food), soda, and refined pastries is critical. Many autism-spectrum children are nutrient deprived and eating toxic food is truly deleterious to their health. I encourage everyone to the watch the documentary entitled "Super Size Me" to see an example of what a fast-food diet can do to you, and your child's health. Other excellent resources are two books – "Fast Food Nation" by Eric Schlosser and "The Crazy Makers" by Carol Simontacchi. You will be amazed, shocked and horrified by what garbage is being promoted by much of the food industry. My advice is to begin making changes to your child's diet right away. Also, incorporating a more healthy diet for everyone in your home will ultimately be beneficial.

I have seen parents spend thousands of dollars on biomedical therapies, tests, and supplements, but fail to make changes in their child's diet. Ultimately, progress is not achieved with their child and parents walk away frustrated that the therapies did not work. You absolutely

MUST start with increased food awareness. You cannot expect to rub on a detoxification cream, take a handful of supplements, get some vitamin shots and expect optimal health for your child if on the back end they are gulping down on a fast food burger with cheese, a side order of fries, sugary cookies, artificial corn chips, milk shakes and/or soda pop 2 to 3 times per day. Be honest with yourself – how much of this type of food does your child get on a daily basis? Weekly?

I know these statements make people uncomfortable and that it is not fashionable to suggest making these sacrifices. Other family members, friends or colleagues may think you are being extreme in making these changes. What they do not realize is that if they eat these foods, their health can become compromised as well. The bottom line is that optimal health will not be achieved if a focus on healthier eating is not a priority. Health is a pursuit – not an event. You have to keep pursuing it for your child. Day after day, as a parent or caregiver, you have to make the choices about what your child will and will not eat – regardless about what anyone else thinks.

There are many resources available with respects to incorporating a nutritious whole food diet. Start exploring your local health food stores or specialty markets for food alternatives that you normally buy at the standard local markets. Incorporating a whole food diet takes time, but is well worth the effort. Be patient and the dividends will pay off with improved health and vitality. Listed are a few resources with regards to improving the quality of food you provide for your child, yourself and family.

- **"Total Health Program"** by Joseph Mercola, D.O. Dr. Mercola's Website at www.mercola.com is an excellent resource for complementary health information.

- **"The Body Ecology Diet"** by Donna Gates www.bodyecologydiet.com. This is a good resource for healthy eating particularly if your child is plagued by recurrent yeast problems.

- **"Nourishing Hope"** by Julie Matthews www.nourishinghope.com. Julie Matthew's is a biomedical nutritionist with years of experience helping parents incorporate healthy eating and special diets.

Dietary Options

Within the biomedical community there are a number of dietary interventions that you will come across including the gluten and casein-free diet (GF/CF), the Specific Carbohydrate Diet (SCD), Low Oxalate Diet (LOD), Feingold, Gut and Psychology Syndrome (GAPS), and anti-candida. All of these diets have their place and unique qualities that make them beneficial for a varying group of children. Deciding on which diet is right for your child can be confusing. How do you know where to start? Which one do I do? Which one is best? All of these are common questions, but sometimes difficult to answer. In my experience there is no one diet that is right for every person. One size does not fit all. What is needed is a brief description of what some these diets are and how they may benefit your child. What you will find overtime is that as you begin with one diet such as the GF/CF you will eventually be incorporating aspects from a variety of diet programs that best suit the needs of your child, lifestyle and family dynamics.

Let's take an example from an eating principle which I feel has a lot of upside – The Body Ecology Diet.

Donna Gates has done a masterful job in putting together a program for reducing foods that stimulate candida (yeast) overgrowth and increasing high quality foods for optimal nutrition. She incorporates a number of food concepts including cultured vegetables, sugar reduction, gluten & casein-free products, and food combining. Here are the highlights of her program:

- Anti-candida diet by eliminating all fruits other than lemons, limes, dried cranberries, and black currant seed juice.
- Cultured vegetables which aide in proper digestion, normalizing intestinal beneficial bacteria levels and acid-alkaline balance.
- Using various kefir products which are a good source of protein.
- Using a wide variety of protein meats, vegetables, and certain non-gluten (gliadin) grains (quinoa, amaranth, millet and buckwheat).
- Vegetable juices for increased nutrient bioavailability.
- Proper food combining to reduce digestive problems such as bloating, gas, and yeast overgrowth.

113

The benefits derived from the Body Ecology program are a reduction in yeast overgrowth (and other opportunistic intestinal "gut bugs" such as bacteria and parasites); reduced exposure to harmful sugars, improved digestion, stronger immune function and less food allergies. What also happens in this dietary program (along with the others that will be described – SCD, Feingold) is that artificial colors (food dyes), flavorings (aspartame, MSG, others), and other harmful ingredients are eliminated.

The need to avoid most fruits is variable for some children depending on how problematic their yeast problems are. The incorporation of grains such as quinoa and amaranth on the Body Ecology Diet may be a slight issue in a highly sensitive child. However, the only way to really know with any of these diets is to begin implementing them and see how your child responds.

The Body Ecology Diet is a good example of how a more whole food diet can have wide-sweeping positive effects by reducing many of the artificial food ingredients, sugars and toxic fats that plague so much of the typical American diet. Let's take a look at a few other common diets used by the biomedical autism community.

Gluten and Casein-Free Diet (GF/CF)

This is the most common diet recommended for children on the autism-spectrum and is usually the first place new parents to the biomedical arena use. It is simply the removal of all gluten (more specifically gliadin) containing grains such as wheat, barley, and rye, as well as cow dairy products containing casein – milk, cheese, commercial yogurts, and ice cream. This diet alone, as reported by the Autism Research Institute and in my clinical experience, has benefited thousands of children with increased speech, better eye contact, improved focusing and attention and digestive function (less loose stools, less gas and bloating). For beginners to the biomedical movement who are just getting started the GF/CF diet is one of the best places to start. There is ample information about how to implement the GF/CF diet even for those on a limited budget.

As part of the GF/CF diet I recommend incorporating soy-free as well. Soy products have a similar chemical structure to that of gluten and casein and for many kids, can be problematic. Some children who continue to suffer with chronic constipation or diarrhea, the avoidance of potatoes, rice and/or corn may be necessary (see Specific Carbohydrate Diet).

With regards to the Gluten-free, Casein-free, and Soy-free diet (GF/CF/SF) there are some good resources you can access to help in the process.

- **"Special Diets for Special Kids"** by Lisa Lewis (Book)
- **"10 Easy Steps for Implementing a Gluten/Casein-Free Diet"** by Mary Romaniec. This handout is also available at www.tacanow.org.
- www.tacanow.org – has additional resource guides and articles for GF/CF diet.
- www.gfcfdiet.com or www.autismndi.com.
- www.AutismActionPlan.com – this is my subscription website for in-depth biomedical information and access to me via the parent forum. As part of this

website there is a 12 Week Action Plan that walks you step-by-step in how to incorporate a GF/CF diet, as well as supportive supplement therapy.

NOTE: It is important to keep in mind that for many children, gluten and casein are not just nuisances that need to be avoided periodically. For many kids, these foods are toxins to their bodies (2). These foods can have adverse chemical effects similar to opiate drugs and can cause chemical addiction in their brains (3). Stop waiting and implement the GF/CF/SF Now. Your child may be one of those kids who respond significantly. You will never know until you try it.

Parents often ask me if they have to do the "The Diet" (meaning the GF/CF and SF diet). My response is, not unless you want to bypass one of the most important and consistently positive therapies I have seen work for children on the autism-spectrum. Is it a "pain in the neck?" Sometimes! Do kids get success with other biomedical therapies without having to be put on the GF/CF diet? Sometimes, but not often! Do not short change your child's health or your potential success in implementing the basics of dietary modification by bypassing this step. You can waste a lot of time and money on other therapies that will not reach their full capacity to work if your child's health is being sabotaged by gluten, casein and/or soy. I recommend a 3 month (preferably 6 months) trial of 100% avoidance. You will generally find that dairy reactions are eliminated fairly quickly (in about 3 to 6 weeks), but gluten can take much longer (3 to 6 months). Soy reactions are usually shorter (about 4 to 8 weeks). In most cases, a 3 month trial is plenty of time to see positive changes.

The GF/CF and soy-free diet (GF/CF/SF) is an area that can create a lot of stress on the part of parents. It takes practice, patience, and perseverance. Some kids respond immediately, some not at all. However, in my experience most kids show positive changes. Unfortunately, there is no magic pill to replace the GF/CF and SF.

The Potential Benefits of Food Desensitization Therapy: NAET, Bioset, and EPD (Enzyme Potentiated Desensitization)

In my clinical experience, certain forms of allergy elimination therapies such as **NAET** www.naet.com or **Bioset** www.bioset-institute.com can help some children reduce their food and environmental allergies and sensitivities to the point were they periodically are able to handle some wheat and dairy in their diet without adverse effects. I have been impressed with these therapies potential. It does not work for all kids, but is certainly worth a try if you can find a qualified practitioner. The principle behind these forms of allergy desensitization techniques (NAET and Bioset) is using acupuncture points that relate to allergy sensitivity and then administering dilute remedies of specific known allergens to short circuit a negative reaction to the particular substance being tested. These treatment sessions are not painful and are safe for children. To learn more about the potential for these therapies and for a health practitioner in your area access the above links.

Another beneficial therapy for children (and adults) with strong negative reactions to foods, food additives and

117

environmental chemicals such as aggression, allergies, headaches, irritability, tantrums, and more is Enzyme Potentiated Desensitization (EPD) as promoted by Doris Rapp, M.D. (www.drrapp.com). Dr. Rapp author of the books "Is This Your Child's World" and "Our Toxic World" has worked for years as an environmental allergy specialist treating patients with physical and behavioral challenges that show strong reactions to environmental pollutants and certain foods.

The Benefits of Digestive Enzymes

Certain digestive enzymes (chemicals in our body that break down food substrate from larger pieces into smaller pieces) seem to help some kids, either by eliminating the need for gluten and casein (and soy) avoidance or diminishing the adverse effects of these foods when accidentally eaten. In my experience, to obtain the full benefit, these enzymes work best if a child has already been on a gluten, casein, and soy-free diet for at least 3 to 6 months. Houston Enzymes are an excellent source of digestive enzymes. **Peptizyde** (chewable forms available) for gluten and casein digestion (digests soy peptides) and **Zyme Prime** (chewable forms available) for protein, fat and carbohydrate digestion are available from New Beginnings Nutritionals at www.nbnus.com or **877-575-2467.** I recommend 1 to 2 capsules (or 2 to 3 chewable tablets) at the beginning of meals. They also carry a combination enzyme product called **TriEnza** which is excellent as well.

Specific Carbohydrate Diet (SCD)

For some children, particularly those with inflammatory bowel conditions (Crohn's Disease, Ulcerative Colitis, Autistic-Enterocolitis); very weak immune systems, or the inability to eradicate opportunistic bacteria and yeast from their digestive systems. They will need to implement a more detailed dietary program. One such program is called the Specific Carbohydrate Diet (SCD) as promoted by the late Elaine Gottschall, author of a groundbreaking book titled **"Breaking the Vicious Cycle"** (www.breakingtheviciouscycle.com). This diet is an extension of the gluten/casein-free diet (and soy-free diet) and has been a big boost for health for many children on the autism-spectrum.

I have seen this diet work miracles with patients with digestive conditions such as Ulcerative Colitis or Crohn's Disease. Many autism children are suffering with a similar condition called Autistic Entereocolitis as described by Andrew Wakefield, M.D. (4). Many more kids are suffering with undiagnosed bowel disorders, and will benefit from the SCD approach.

The SCD is not just a low carbohydrate diet, but instead is focused on removing certain grains such as wheat, barley, rye (same as the GF/CF diet), as well as rice, corn and other offending foods. The theory is that certain digestive enzymes that breakdown disaccharides (complex sugars) are missing (or are being blocked from reaching the food in the digestive system by excessive layers of intestinal mucus) in the child's digestive system making it difficult to digest these additional

119

food sources. The lack of proper digestive function leads to chronic inflammation in the digestive system which contributes to gut wall deterioration. With the breakdown of the gut wall food absorption becomes compromised leading to mineral, amino acid and vitamin imbalances, as well as immune dysfunction and the overgrowth of opportunistic infections such as yeast and bacteria.

The digestive system is the largest immune organ in the body and acts as the first line immune defense against pathogens such as parasites, yeast, bacteria and intestinal exposed viruses. The loss of this immune response and the eventually breakdown of the gut wall can lead to systemic immune dysfunction and leaky gut. Leaky gut is analogous to a screen door on a submarine – "everything and anything can get through." This means you lose the ability to keep the bad stuff from entering your blood stream. Increased toxins filtering into your child's blood stream can activate systemic immune responses leading to local and systemic inflammation – including the brain (5). Celiac disease (which is a genetic disorder evidenced by the inability to digest gluten – specifically gliadin – containing grains) is an example where gluten proteins from food can adversely affect the brain.

One chemical that can become engaged in the process of a hyperimmune response is Tumor Necrosis Factor – alpha (TNF-a) which is a contributor to digestive and neurological inflammation in autism (6). TNF-a is found elevated in other neurological disorders such as Multiple Sclerosis, Lou Gehrig's Disease (ALS), and even HIV-AIDS. In AIDS it is felt that too much TNF-α contributes to the "wasting syndrome" that eventually weakens the individual to the point where they are overcome with opportunistic infections.

Some parents choose to implement the SCD at the same time as the standard GF/CF diet. For many in the autism biomedical community, the feeling is the SCD is far superior to the GF/CF approach for long-term benefit for the child. With everything, there is a balance that needs to be struck. I have personally seen the SCD work wonders for many children – improved language, eye contact, attention, etc. However, some kids can tend to have some issues with the SCD over a period of time, such as increased ammonia production from too much protein if the diet is not well balanced or a continuation of yeast overgrowth in the beginning stages by not avoiding enough fruit and simple sugars (which is what the Body Ecology Diet advocates). Also, some kids develop too much oxalates (discussed below) which can contribute to aggressive behavior, irritability, and sleeping issues. Even though these two conditions are not something I have seen as a major problem for many kids doing the SCD it is something to watch out for.

- **Ammonia Issues** – the SCD by nature can be a high protein diet because of the elimination of certain grains. This in itself is not a problem, but some children tend to have problems eliminating ammonia. Ammonia is a byproduct of protein metabolism. A fair amount of children will have tendency to produce ammonia in their digestive systems because of imbalances in intestinal bacteria and yeast or metabolically in their body because of certain biochemical and genetic factors. The end result is increased self-stimulatory behavior – usually hand-flapping, but some kids lose focus, become lethargic, agitated and lack attention. In hospitals ammonia is measured in patients with chronic liver disorders – particularly liver failure. At extremely high levels ammonia can be lethal. In the autism community we are not talking about lethal levels of ammonia. Instead, we are relating it to low level imbalances that can affect a child's cognitive function.

Ammonia levels can be checked via a standard blood test. A urine amino acid test can give an indication of ammonia as well, but this tool can be problematic because the level of ammonia can be influenced by decay of the urine sample if not refrigerated properly.

- **Oxalates** – oxalates are organic compounds found in many vegetables (spinach, swiss chard, sweet potatoes), nuts (almonds, peanuts), fruits (rhubarb, various berries), and other foods. These can cause problems with respects to generalized inflammation if too high in the diet. Oxalates in the diet are generally bound to calcium and eliminated via the stool. However, with prolonged intestinal damage from ongoing food sensitivities, yeast and bacteria overgrowth high oxalates can be absorbed into the blood stream and generate systemic inflammation. See the next section for a more in-depth discussion regarding oxalates.

Low Oxalate Diet (LOD)

As we discussed, oxalates (and its acid form called oxalic acid) are organic compounds primarily found in many different types of food. However, there are a few other sources as well – aspergillus and penicillium molds (7), as well as genetic disorders of oxalate metabolism.

Oxalates for most of us are naturally occurring compounds that reach our digestive system through food and are harmlessly broken down by the abundance of naturally occurring lactic acid bacteria and eliminated in our feces. The problem occurs when these bacteria, particularly one called Oxalobacter formigens (8) are destroyed by antibiotics or other intestinal toxins. When this occurs the oxalates in food are not digested properly and can be absorbed unopposed into our blood stream. Here they can interact with essential minerals such as zinc, calcium and magnesium. For some individuals the formation of kidneys stones – primarily calcium oxalate stones is the result. However, oxalate crystals have been shown to accumulate in other body tissues including the joints, muscle tissue and brain.

Oxalates can even bind heavy metals such as mercury, lead, and cadmium inside cells preventing them from being excreted effectively. Susan Owens (an independent biomedical researcher) has done a tremendous amount of work on the oxalate issue and is helping parents incorporate what is called the Low Oxalate Diet (LOD) as a specialized program to meet some of the ongoing challenges ASD kids may have.

Susan has reported, based on her tracking of parent responses through her Yahoo! Support group called **Trying Low Oxalates** that some kids benefit in the following ways:

- Improvement in gross and fine motor skills
- Improvement in expressive speech
- Increased imitation skills
- Increased sociability
- Decreased rigidity
- Improved sleep
- Reduced self-abusive behavior
- Loss of bed wetting
- Loss of frequent urination
- Improvement in anemia
- …and many more

Dr. William Shaw from the Great Plains Laboratory has put together a useful handout regarding the issue about oxalates and autism at www.greatplainslaboratory.com, and his ongoing research shows that oxalates are a definite issue with some kids on the autism-spectrum. It is a possibility that continued yeast problems seen with many children is a stimulus for some of their oxalate abundance which brings the need for continued anti fungal (anti yeast) treatment into the mix.

You can access more information about oxalates from Susan Owen's website at www.lowoxalate.info.

Feingold Program, Phenol and Salicylate Sensitivity

This category of dietary intervention holds a tremendous amount of promise for many children on the autism-spectrum, as well as those with Attention Deficit (ADD) and Attention Deficit Hyperactivity Disorder (ADHD). Here, I will briefly discuss what these items mean and resources you can access to get more specific information.

The basic upshot of this segment is that many children on the autism-spectrum have difficulty with sulfur chemistry (9) which is important for the processing of naturally occurring food chemicals called phenols and other substances called salicylates (which are a group of chemicals related to aspirin). When these food chemicals are ingested, they can trigger a host of behavioral problems including hyperactivity, agitation, irritability, violent behavior and others. The Feingold Program (www.feingold.org) is a dietary elimination procedure to determine if certain foods and food additives (and non-food items such as fragrances) contribute to a child's behavior problems.

Feingold Program

Ben F. Feingold, M.D. was a pediatrician and Chief of Allergy at Kaiser-Permanente Medical Center in San Francisco, CA in the 1960's. For years, he had been using a diet that eliminated aspirin and aspirin-like foods (salicylates) for patients with asthma and skin conditions (10) with good success. When he started to remove synthetic colorings and flavorings from people's diets, they also showed dramatic improvement. Shortly thereafter, a patient of Dr. Feingold who was being treated for a mood disorder began to show dramatic improvement while using his new diet for her hive condition. He began recommending this diet to other patients as well, including many pediatric patients, not only with skin conditions, but hyperactivity. The results were that these kids got better. Over the years, this dietary program has been modified, but today remains a very beneficial program for parents to try with their children who are suffering with asthma, allergies, eczema and other skin conditions, as well as behavioral problems including hyperactivity (11). The basic overview of the Feingold Program eliminates the following additives:

- Artificial Colorings (synthetic, i.e. "man-made")
- Artificial Flavorings (synthetic, i.e. "man-made")
- Aspartame (Nutrasweet), MSG
- Artificial preservatives: BHA, BHT, TBHQ

More information about the specifics of the Feingold Program can be obtained from the Feingold Institute at www.feingold.org.

Phenol Sensitivity

Phenols are chemicals found in many different foods. These are naturally occurring chemicals that are found abundantly in nature, including our own bodies. It is impossible to eliminate phenols 100% from your child's diet, as they are found in many foods known to be nutritious – almonds, apples, apricots, berries, cherries, cloves, grapes, oranges, peaches, tomatoes and more. Phenol chemicals can also be synthetic, such as artificial colorings and flavorings. Phenols should be thought of as a group of chemicals, both food and non-food. One subgroup is salicylates,which was researched and eliminated through the Feingold Program. In fact, when you implement the Feingold Program, you are essentially eliminating a group of phenols items from your child's diet.

Rosemary Waring, Ph.D has described a condition seen commonly in ASD children called phenol-sulfutransferase deficiency, or PST (see reference paper 9 titled "Sulfur Metabolism in Autism"). This is an enzyme found in the liver that deactivates phenol subgroups through the chemical interaction with sulfur. Sulfur is an abundant chemical in our body needed for a host of chemical processes related to detoxification. Many children have a PST deficiency leading to a difficulty in processing phenols. Here is a list of common symptoms seen with phenol sensitivity (hint: these same symptoms can be seen with a person with salicylate sensitivity and improved through the Feingold program):

- Aggression
- Diarrhea
- Frequent night waking
- Headache
- Head-banging (or other self-injurious behavior)
- Hyperactivity
- Inappropriate laughter ("goofy, giddy and silly" – similar to what is seen with candida)
- Poor sleep

The goal with phenol reduction is not to eliminate all phenol foods, but to significantly reduce your child's exposure. As time goes on they become healthier and more tolerant, particularly of the natural phenol foods. You will have to explore what works for your particular child and become a detective with what types of foods seem to cause them problems. Some parents have found success using the phenol digestive enzymes which help to breakdown and neutralize excess phenols in the diet. One particular product I like is from Houston Enzymes called **No-Fenol**. This can be obtained from New Beginnings at www.nbnus.com - 1 to 2 capsules (or 2 to 3 chewable tablets) with a known high phenol containing food is generally recommended.

So Where to Begin

In this chapter, we've explored a number of different dietary options to consider for your child. It isn't always easy to figure out which one to implement first or where to begin. Here are some general recommendations:

1. If you are brand new to biomedical information and you are feeling overwhelmed with all the information – start with the basics. Begin the gluten and casein-free diet first. The article titled "Going GFCF in 10 weeks" is an excellent place to start. **Again, www.AutismActionPlan.com has the 12 Week Action Plan which is a step-by-step guide through GF/CF diet implementation.**

2. If your child continues to suffer with chronic loose stools (and you have done the appropriate testing for digestive infections – see Chapter 8) than introducing the Specific Carbohydrate Diet (SCD) is likely necessary.

3. If you feel your child regressed after an MMR vaccine (or others) and continues to suffer with bowel

problems, the SCD is most likely going to be needed over just the GF/CF (and soy-free diet).

4. If your child is hyperactive or shows signs of aggression, irritability, tantrums, or other symptoms related to phenol sensitivity, incorporation of the Feingold Program is going to be useful.

Hint:

If you implement the SCD program, you will start to reduce many of the artificial colors and flavorings as well. This does not always happen when doing a basic GF/CF diet because kids can still be exposed to a lot of artificial products.

5. If yeast and intestinal bacteria continues to be a problem with little or no resolution from anti-fungal (anti-yeast) therapy, then a more strict anti-candida program is warranted. The Body Ecology Diet is one option for this. Remember, this diet eliminates a lot of fruit, but allows some grains that the SCD program may frown upon at first. However, the upside is that it all but eliminates the artificial colorings and flavoring which are problematic for phenol sensitive kids.

6. The Low Oxalate Diet may become necessary if your child continues to deal with poor attention, decreased fine and gross motor function, poor social skills, bed-wetting and/or frequent urination. If there is a family history of kidney stones, the LOD would be something to consider sooner than later. Also, oxalates appear from clinical experience to increase the

sensitivity to phenol foods, so the LOD can overtime help with phenol sensitivity as well.

My advice – be patient! Learning to implement one of these diets or synchronizing facets of these diets takes time, self-education, and preparation. It's all about educating yourself and beginning the process. As you become more knowledgeable, the principles behind these diets becomes easier. You start to see patterns and understand how your child responds.

Ultimately, your child is the best barometer of how these diets may work. There are no quick fixes. Every child responds differently. Usually patterns are consistent – better eye contact, more focusing and attention, fewer tantrums, aggressive, and self-abusive behavior. Kids become healthier and their digestive systems work better with more formed stools, less bloating, gas and diarrhea/constipation. They look healthier, are more engaged socially and seem genuinely happier, but this takes time.

From my experience the incorporation of dietary changes is the single most important thing you can do for your child. Without a healthier diet – optimal health will not be achieved. The road to autism recovery or overall improvement will be almost impossible without a healthy diet.

References:

(1) Elder JH. The gluten-free, casein-free diet in autism: an overview with clinical implications. *Nutr Clin Pract.*2008 Dec-2009 Jan;23(6):583-8.

(2) Vojdani A, O'Bryan T, Green JA, Mccandless J, Woeller KN, Vojdani E, Nourian AA, Cooper EL. Immune response to dietary proteins, gliadin and cerebellar peptides in children with autism. *Nutr Neurosci.* 2004 Jun; 7(3):151-61

(3) Adams JB, et al. The severity of autism is associated with toxic metal body burden and red blood cell glutathione levels. *J Toxicol.* 2009;2009:532640.

(4) Hsu CL, Lin CY, Chen CL, Wang CM, Wong MK. The effects of a gluten and casein-free diet in children with autism: a case report. *Chang Gung Med J.* 2009 Jul-Aug; 32(4):459-65.

(5) Wakefield AJ et al. Enterocolitis in children with developmental disorders. *Am J Gastroenterol.* 2000 Sep; 95(9):2285-95.

(6) (Jyonouchi H, et al. Evaluation of an association between gastrointestinal symptoms and cytokine production against common dietary proteins in children with autism spectrum disorders. *J Pediatr.* 2005 May;146(5): 605-10.

(7) (Jyonouchi H, Sun S, Le H. Proinflammatory and regulatory cytokine production associated with innate and adaptive immune re-sponses in children with autism spectrum disorders and developmental regression. *J Neuroimmunol.* 2001 Nov 1;120(1-2):170-9.

(8) Lee SH, Barnes WG, Schaetzel WP. Pulmonary aspergillosis and the importance of oxalate crystal

recognition in cytology specimens. Arch Pathol Lab Med. 1986.

(9) Kumar R, Mukherjee M, Bhandari M, Kumar A, Sidhu H, Mittal RD. Role of Oxalobacter formigenes in calcium oxalate stone disease: a study from North India. Eur Urol. 2002 Mar;41(3):318-22.

(10) Waring RH, Klovrza LV. Sulphur metabolism in autism. *J Nutr Env Med*. 2000;10:25-32.

(11) Michaelsson G, Juhlin L. <u>Urticaria induced by preservatives and dye additives in food and drugs.</u>, *Br J Dermatol* 1973 Jun;88(6):525-32

(12) Kamel MM, El-lethey HS. The Potential Health Hazard of Tartrazine and Levels of Hyperactivity, Anxiety-Like Symptoms, Depression and Anti-social behaviour in Rats. *Journal of American Science*, 2011;7(6)

Chapter 9

The Use of Methylcobalamin (MB-12) Therapy to Support Methylation Problems in in Autism-Spectrum Children

This is one of the most important therapies that I use in my practice. I have seen more positive things occur with this one treatment alone over the years, particularly in the <u>early</u> stages of biomedical treatment, than with many other therapies. I define "early" as the first 4 to 8 weeks. As we discussed in Chapter 6 "Implementing the Action Plan," I feel you must start building the foundation for good health with proper diet, basic supplements, and diagnostic testing to create a launching point for biomedical success for your child. Methycobalamin (aka. Methyl-B12 or MB-12) is a therapy that helps in my experience over 90% of those on the autism-spectrum - both children and adults. This doesn't mean that it is a panacea or "magic bullet" for all cases of autism. However, it has wide-sweeping effects with respect to speech, attentiveness, environmental awareness, and better mental and emotional stability.

To understand the benefits of this therapy it is important that you have some idea of how Methyl-B12 works. To understand the true biochemical underpinnings of most cases of autism you need to understand the chemistry of methylation and Methyl-B12. Yes, I know I told you that you would not have to become a biochemist, but it is still worth trying to understand a little about how this nutrient functions in the body. Let me briefly explain a very important system called Methylation. This biochemical process is essential in life and plays a HUGE role in the overall treatment of autism (1).

What is Methylation?

Methylation is a biochemical process that supports the cardiovascular, hormone, immune, detoxification, DNA/ RNA structure and functions, plus other key metabolic systems. There are some very effective therapies that support this reaction, namely methylcobalamin (injection, nasal, oral), as well as other methylating supplements such as dimethylglycine (DMG) and trimethylglycine (TMG). However, according to James Neubrander, M.D., the pioneer in MB-12 injection therapy - the subcutaneous injection route is the most effective (article titled - "Methyl-B12: Myth, Masterpiece, or Miracle"). This has also been my experience.

The Genetics of Methylation Problems in Autistic Individuals

The most commonly studied and referenced chemical reactions in this methylation system are re-methylation and trans-sulfuration.

◆ **Re-Methylation (or methylation)** - this pathway involves the conversion of homocysteine to methionine. Production of methionine (see #1 in diagram below), an amino acid, is the rate-limiting step (rate limiting = nothing can move faster in a biochemical process) for the conversion of other necessary chemicals that affect the heart and blood vessels, muscle tissue, immune and nervous systems. The conversion of homocysteine to methionine can occur by direct transference of a methyl (CH3) groups from methylcobalamin (B12) or betaine (trimethylglycine or TMG)

Homocysteine sits at a junction of two different biochemical reactions. Because of its position in this biochemical matrix it has the capacity to impact methylation and sulfur group transference processes in the body. A risk factor for elevated homocysteine is *increased risk* for cardiovascular disease (2). However, in children with autism a faulty methylation system affects other functions as well, particularly cognitive areas including concentration, attention (3), and language development.

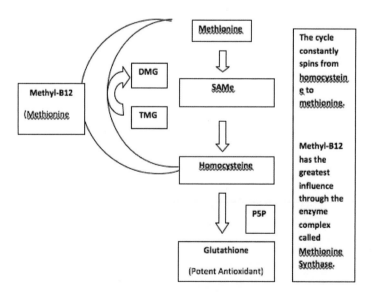

♦ **Trans-Sulfuration** - this pathway involves converting homocysteine into two different amino acids - taurine and cysteine. Taurine is most commonly known for heart and liver support, detoxification, bile acid formation, and cholesterol excretion. Cysteine has a direct influence on glutathione production.

Glutathione is a potent antioxidant and has protective effects against DNA/RNA damage, as well as being involved in heavy metal and chemical detoxification and immune function. Many children on the autism-spectrum have dysfunctions with regards to taurine and cysteine regulation (4).

There are many intermediary steps involved in these two biochemical reactions. It is important to keep the big picture in mind when referencing these pathways. Envision a wheel that is constantly spinning in a clockwise direction. Homocysteine is at 6 o'clock and Methionine is at 12 o'clock. The goal is to get from 6 o'clock to 12 o'clock and then from 12 o'clock to 6 o'clock. Other chemicals will impact this wheel at specific points. If any one of these intermediary steps is blocked, then the wheel slows down causing biochemical imbalance. This causes a backlog of chemical information that has deleterious effects on other dependent systems such as immune system regulation, hormone production, detoxification capacity, and DNA structure and function.

Methylcobalamin (MB-12), Folic Acid (more specifically Folinic Acid or Methyl-Folate), and Betaine (TMG) are responsible for adding proper conversion of homocysteine from 6 o'clock to methionine at 12 o'clock. SAMe

136

(s-adenosylmethionine), the body's "universal methyl donor," helps take methionine from 12 o'clock back to homocysteine at the 6 o'clock position.

The issue with many autism-spectrum children is that this system does not operate properly. This has an enormous negative impact on their health, such as increased susceptibility to chronic infections, inability to detoxify chemicals and heavy metals, and neurocognitive problems such as language processing, attention, and concentration. Genetic susceptibility certainly plays a role. However, for many the problem does not manifest itself until a child's system is negatively impacted by nutritional deficiencies, digestive problems from yeast, bacteria, parasites, malabsorption from digestive inflammation, chemical pollutants, and heavy metal toxins, such as mercury from vaccines or environmental exposures.

Methylcobalamin (MB-12) Therapy – The Gold Standard Approach

The gold standard approach at this time (from clinical experience) is MB-12 given by subcutaneous (under the skin) injection. Injections are given in the buttocks every three days using a pre-filled insulin syringe and needle. It's virtually painless. If some stinging does occur, with a prescription you can get a numbing agent like EMLA (lidocaine) cream from your local pharmacy. Some pharmacies carry over-the-counter numbing creams as well, i.e. LMX topical numbing cream. Most numbing creams have a lidocaine substance which numbs the skin. Apply the cream onto the skin prior to the injection as directed to reduce sensitivity from the injection. You can also use this numbing cream before blood draws as well.

The most difficult part of the process of MB-12 injection therapy is for you as the parent to overcome your fear of giving the injection. Yes! That's right - Mom, Dad, Grandma or Grandpa – whomever will be giving the injection will need to get over their apprehension. Luckily there are very good instructions available for performing this procedure. Instructions for "dispensing and disposal" of MB-12 can be found from Dr. Neubrander's website at www.drneubrander.com. You can also obtain detailed information on the application of Methyl-B12 from my biomedical subscription website at www.AutismActionPlan.com in the "Methyl-B12" section.

If you are going to ask your personal physician for a prescription for MB-12, then making it as simple as possible for them will benefit everyone. Unfortunately, you cannot go to your local pharmacy and get the right type of Methyl-B12 (it is different from the common vitamin B12) that I am describing in the book (unless your specific pharmacy has taken the time to learn how to process methylcobalamin injections as outlined by Dr. Neubrander. Listed within the **"Any Physician Can Order Methyl-B12"** section are four pharmacies I commonly use for MB-12. They provide Methyl-B12 in the correct concentration and with the correct syringes.

NOTE: My recommendation is *not* to try to shortcut this process by using a brand from your local pharmacy, unless you absolutely know that they have the specifics for compounding Methyl-B12 according to Dr. Neubrander. If your local pharmacist wants to learn how to prepare it correctly they can get the information from www.drneubrander.com.

What Are the Benefits You Can Expect From Methyl-B12 Injections?

- With the use of MB-12 many children improve in three general areas:

    ○ **Cerebral Cortex Function** – develop higher cognitive awareness such as better attention, as well as improved focusing and mental processing skills. Often, kids become better at following commands and more aware of their surroundings.
    ○ **Speech and Language Function** – develop better capacity to speak – many times spontaneously; improved receptive and expressive language, and more complex speech and sentence structure.
    ○ **Emotion and Socialization Function** – develop improved social skills including willingness to socialize, playfulness, appropriate play, interested in other people, as well gaining more emotional stability.

Any Physician Can Order Methyl-B12

- Any physician can order MB-12. All that is needed is a willingness to do so, and the knowledge of how to write the prescription. At the end of this section on

MB-12 injections is an example of how a common prescription for MB-12 is written.

- Once a prescription is sent to the pharmacy they will send you pre-filled syringes with the amount of MB-12 needed for your child at each dose. They supply the exact amount based on your child's weight from a concentration solution of 25mg/ml. This is necessary to achieve the therapeutic benefits of MB-12 therapy according to Dr. Neubrander's research.

- The pharmacy provides MB-12 in pre-filled Becton Dickinson 3/10cc insulin syringes, item #328438. If your personal physician is ordering these for the first time it is wise for them to be specific about syringe size and item number. The four pharmacies that I commonly use for MB-12 prescriptions – **Hopewell (800-792-6670), Lee-Silsby Pharmacy (800-918-8831), Park Pharmacy (866-551-7195)** and **Wellness Pharmacy (800-227-2627)** – are already aware of the specifics needed to provide MB-12 the correct way. For more information about other pharmacies offering Methyl-B12 injections see Dr. Neubrander's website at www.drneubrander.com.

Methyl-B12 Dosing Specifics and Instructions

This section is specific for dosing instructions and how to administer the injections properly. It can be used by physicians looking to provide Methyl-B12 injection therapy:

- The dose is based on a child's weight in kilograms (kg), which is the weight in pounds divided by 2.2 (Example: 150 lbs/2.2=70 kg). The dose of MB-12 at 64.5 mcg is then multiplied by the number of Kg. Thus, 64.5 mcg x 70 kg = 4515 mcg per dose which rounded off becomes 4500 mcg per pre-filled syringe. The dosing of MB-12 is usually done in 250 mcg doses. Each 0.01cc equals 250 mcg from a base concentration of 25 mg/ml (or 25,000 micrograms/millimeter). Thus, on average a 40 lbs child (18 kilograms) would receive a 1250 mcg (or 0.05cc) dose.

- The injection must be given in the subcutaneous fat of the buttocks. Other "fat" areas, such as the abdomen, deltoids (shoulder) do *not* give the same effect. A 30 degree angle or **less** is best and will ensure that the medicine is not given into the child's muscle which can cause the MB-12 to be wasted by being circulated too quickly through the body.

- As stated above the prescription can be sent by your local physician to a certified pharmacy for #10 pre-filled syringes (some doctor's give #15 or #20 to start). I generally recommend starting with 10 syringes, and then following up with your physician 2 to 3 weeks after you start MB-12. At this point a refill can be sent for more. This initial supply will last 30 days (with an expiration date of approximately 60 days). In the beginning give the injection every **72 hours** (every 3 days).

Other Recommendations

- I recommend that other biomedical changes, such as beginning heavy metal detoxification, dietary changes, or new supplements NOT be started during the first 6 weeks of MB-12 shots. If you have already started some of those therapies then it is best to avoid making any other changes during the first six weeks of MB-12.

- Ideally, TMG, DMG or Folinic Acid (or Methyl-Folate) should *not* be started at the same time as MB-12 (during the first 6 weeks). These supplements have been known to increase the potential onset of side effects if started too early. See the section on side effects for more details. If your child is taking DMG (and is tolerating it just fine) it's okay to continue using it – watch however for increased side effects, i.e. hyperness, stimming. If taking TMG, I recommend it be discontinued when starting MB-12 for the first 6 weeks.

- Most children respond favorably during the first six weeks of treatment. They can have increased eye contact and environmental awareness, improved language and social interactions. However, some take longer to respond. I recommend they continue this therapy for at least 12 to 24 months. The average time in my practice is approximately 15 to 18 months.

- About 60 to 70% of the children respond favorably during the first six weeks. Another 5-10% can take a little longer. Responding favorably means more positive changes are happening that are obvious to you. Approximately, 15 - 20% of children are more subtle in their response and it is not until the "Parent Designed Report Form" is filled out (www.drneubrander.com) that positive changes are recognized. This form is filled out at the end of the first six weeks of MB-12 therapy. A minimal number of children do not show any positive changes during the initial phase of MB-12 therapy. However, I still feel that a parent needs to use MB-12 injections for at least a minimum of 15 weeks -- preferably longer to see if positive changes will happen. I know this is a considerable time commitment, but you just *do not* want to miss out on the benefits of this important therapy.

What Are the Common Side Effects From Methyl-B12 Injections?

- Dr. Neubrander reports that side effects such as hyperactivity, increased stimming, disrupted sleep patterns, and mouthing objects are the most common manifestations of negative reactions to MB-12. It is reported that if these side effects are seen the parents who "push through" with the therapy report that the effects eventually lessen and their children greatly improve. This too has been my experience. These side effects may last anywhere between 2 to 6 months. In my experience 4 to 6 weeks is more common.

- All side effects should be classified as tolerable versus intolerable. Take hyperactivity for example. A tolerable side effect of hyperactivity may be that your child is more hyperactive at home, but in their therapy sessions they are more focused, or they are more sociable, and have better eye contact. An intolerable side effect of hyperactivity could be if your child begins "bouncing off the walls" 24/7, and that they cannot focus their attention at all – a pattern that is disruptive in their ability to learn and function.

- Another fairly common side effect is sleep interference. This does not mean complete insomnia, but instead a restless or "fidgety" sleep. This usually resolves in four to six weeks. Mouthing of objects like putting toys or fingers in the mouth occurs in about 30% of the kids. Sometimes they will chew or gnaw on their knuckles. This reaction is short-lived and in most cases is easy to re-direct. The best guess as to why this is happening is nerve activation in the mouth and the child is drawn to mouth objects.

- None of these side effects are life-threatening. I have never seen liver, kidney, or neurological damage from MB-12. Overall, this has been an extremely safe and very effective treatment.

RECAP:

This information can be given to your local physician for ordering the Methyl-B12 injections:

- Ask your physician to write a prescription for Methylcobalamin Injections in the following manner:

Methylcobalamin Injection

_____ mcg per dose of 25mg/ml concentration

using BD 3/10 cc Insulin Syringe, item #328438

#10 Pre-Filled Syringes

Inject SQ q 3 days

- This prescription can be faxed to one of the pharmacies listed previously.
- SQ = subcutaneous (underneath the skin in the subcutaneous fat) and q 3 days = every 3 days (72 hours)

Chapter 10

Stimulation of Monoamine Oxidase-A (MAO-A)
by
Respen-A™ as a Treatment Option for Individuals with an Autism-Spectrum Disorder

By Elaine DeLack, R.N.

"Since 2009 I have been using a therapy called Respen-A in my practice. Respen-A is reported (as you will learn in the article by Elaine DeLack, R.N.) to assist with serotonin metabolism which improves core issues in autism, such as socialization and language problems, sensory system issues, and behavioral imbalances. As you will see this therapy holds a tremendous amount of potential for helping many individuals on the autism-spectrum. I am introducing this information about Respen-A here because I believe it important for you to understand. This chapter, although more technical in nature than previous chapters in this book, explains in detail how Respen-A works and the benefits often seen.

My overall impression with Respen-A is that it is an extremely useful biomedical treatment option for the vast majority who try it, and has become an important part of my treatment approach for autism as its beneficial effects are often seen shortly after starting it. It is not uncommon to have parents report better behavior, improved language skills, and increased social engagement within a few short weeks of starting Respen-A. in my opinion it deserves serious consideration as a primary biomedical intervention similar to how the autism biomedical community views the gluten and casein-free diet, dietary supplements, anti-yeast treatment and Methyl-B12 therapy" – Dr. Woeller

146

Monoamine oxidase-A (MAO-A) is genetically expressed on the X chromosome as either a high activity allele or a low activity allele. Low activity alleles within the gene promoter region of the MAO-A gene were correlated in autistic patients (1, 2). Individuals with the low activity allele MAO-A gene polymorphism display behaviors of alcoholism, antisocial personality, and impulsivity (3, 4) and aggressive behaviors have been associated with decreased MAO-A activity (5). Autistic patients often exhibit impulsivity, aggression, and antisocial behaviors.

The possible causal relationship of decreased MAO-A activity results in the core symptoms of ASD has not been investigated to date using placebo controlled double blind studies. A study conducted by Edward Lehman, MD, Joseph Haber, MD, and Stanley Lesser, MD was published in 1957 in The Journal of Nervous and Mental Disease. High doses of reserpine (a potent stimulator of MAO-A activity (6, 7) were administered orally for 5-7 months to 9 children, ages 3 ½ to 9 years, who had been diagnosed with severe autism. This study was not blinded and it did not have a placebo control group. Despite the limitations of the small study, all 9 of the children showed improvement in interaction with the environment and others, improved pattern of play, increased ability to communicate on a nonverbal level, and increased willingness to eat a larger variety of foods and textures (8). But, the higher doses of reserpine in these children also had a tranquilizing effect and toxic symptoms appeared in 4 children.

More recent anecdotal data collected from Autism Treatment Evaluation Checklist (ATEC) evaluations completed by the parents of patients using a transdermal low dose of reserpine via the topical disc called Respen-A™ revealed an average 19 points of improvement in the total ATEC score which correlated with 30% improvement in the overall total scores and a statistical significance of $p \leq 0.00002$. This was an N of 23, comprised of 19 boys and 4 girls, ages ranged from 2-33 years of age with a baseline total ATEC score of 25-108 (only one patient had a baseline score less than 30). The reserpine was administered in 0.01 mg doses once a day for up to one year duration. The Figure 1a and 1b illustrate the results of this anecdotal data.

Figure 1a

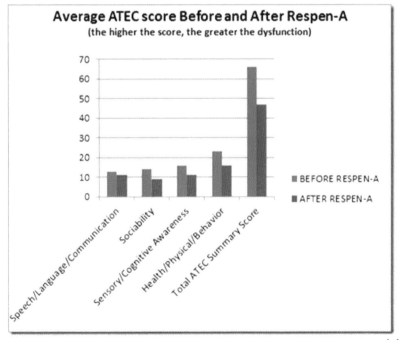

Figure 1b

CORE SYMPTOM EVALUATED	BEFORE RESPEN-A	AFTER RESPEN-A	Significance	% of Mean Improvement
Speech/Language/ Communication	13	11	P = 0.001	18%
Sociability	14	9	P = 0.002	32%
Sensory/Cognitive Awareness	16	11	P = 0.0004	32%
Health/Physical/Behavior	23	16	P = 0.0004	33%
Total ATEC Summary Score	66	47	P = 0.00002	30%

Scientific Rationale Behind Respen-A™

The significant improvement in the core symptoms of ASD with the stimulation of MAO-A using Respen-A™ lends the question, "Could a deficiency in the activity of MAO-A explain many of the metabolic imbalances associated with ASD?"

MAO-A is an enzyme expressed in the brain that metabolizes histamine, serotonin, norepinephrine, and to a lesser extent dopamine (Dopamine is predominantly metabolized by MAO-B). High levels of serotonin (hyperserotonemia) and high levels of norepinephrine are associated with ASD (10, 11). Oxytocin is involved in the development of social and language communication skills. Deficient oxytocin innervation has been postulated as a potential contributor to the development of ASD. In a developmental

149

hyperserotonemia model of autism in Sprague-Dawley rats, pregnant dams were administered a serotonin agonist. The dams' offspring displayed decreased bonding with the dam, increased gnawing reactions to novel stimulus, less behavioral inhibition, and had fewer olfactory-based social interactions. Post mortem analyses revealed a loss of oxytocin containing cells in the paraventricular nucleus of the hypothalamus in the pups that had been exposed to high levels of serotonin during gestation (12). Thus, the decrease in oxytocin associated with ASD may be in part due to high levels of serotonin as a result of decreased MAO-A activity.

Serotonin is a mediator of the hypothalamic-pituitary-adrenal (HPA) axis. Serotonin's regulation of the HPA axis is mediated via activation of the various serotonin receptors. The secretion of adrenocorticotropic hormone (ACTH) is mediated via the 5-HT1a, 5-HT2a, and 5-HT2c receptors (14). Serotonin that has not been metabolized by MAO-A will be transported by the serotonin reuptake transporter to the 5-HT1a receptors (15, 16, 17). This stimulation of the 5-HT1a receptor results in increased ACTH secretion that is seen in ASD (18). Catechol-O-methyltransferase (COMT) can also stimulate ACTH secretion but this is dependent on low-expression MAO-A variant in the same individual (19).

ASD patients have a slowed response to stress despite elevated levels of ACTH (20). MAO-A knockout mice have demonstrated a diminished response to stress (21). Chronic stress in persons with low activity MAO-A alleles display a pattern of cortisol excretion - a decrease from overnight to daytime - that is suggestive of HPA axis blunting as compared to those persons with more active MAO-A alleles (22). Children with infantile autism have shown an abnormal diurnal rhythm for cortisol production (23).

Increased levels of serotonin stimulates the release of hypothalamic corticotropin-releasing hormone (CRH), increases ACTH secretion 3-5 fold and increases secretion of proopiomelanocortin hormone (POMC) 15-27%, all of which have been shown to be elevated in ASD (24). POMC stimulates the production of Beta-endorphins, which has been shown to be high in many autistic patients especially those who display self-injurious behavior (25). MAO-A is a mitochondrial enzyme present in the brain, liver, pancreas and adrenal glands. Mitochondria complex I, II, III, IV, and V dysfunction is associated with ASD (9). A decrease in the MAO-A activity can decrease the mitochondrial complex II activity (reduced flavin adenine dinucleotide (FADH)) as it is dependent on the MAO-A activity (26). Inhibition of mitochondrial complex II results in an accumulation of dopamine's metabolite HVA (27). HVA is elevated in ASD patients (28). Tryptophan is metabolized to serotonin which is then metabolized by MAO-A into 5-Hydroxyindoleacetaldehyde (5-HIAL) which is the physiologically active metabolite of serotonin. The 5-HIAL is then metabolized into 5-Hydroxyindoleacetic acid (5-HIAA) which is the excreted metabolite of serotonin. If the MAO-A is deficient resulting in the buildup of serotonin, the majority of the tryptophan is then metabolized via the kynurenine pathway resulting in quinolinic acid. Organic Acid Tests on patients with ASD often show high quinolinic acid and low 5-HIAA and a high quinolinic:5-HIAA ratio.

151

Quinolinic acid at high levels is a neurotoxin. Brain toxicity due to high quinolinic acid has been implicated in Alzheimer's, autism, Huntington's disease, stroke, dementia from old age, depression, HIV related dementia, and schizophrenia. A high quinolinic acid to 5-HIAA ratio indicates excessive inflammation and excessive cortisol production, both of which are present in ASD (31).

ASD patients such as those with Asperger Syndrome have elevated total cholesterol and low-density lipoprotein (LDL) levels (29). Higher total cholesterol, LDL/HDL ratios, and triglycerides were associated with low activity MAO-A alleles (30). It is also reported that several autism patients have abnormally low total cholesterol. A possible explanation for this, despite having low MAO-A activity, may be the decreased MAO-A:MAO-B ratio. Monoamine oxidase exists in two forms, MAO-A and MAO-B. As stated previously, MAO-A metabolizes histamine, serotonin and norepinephrine, whereas MAO-B metabolizes only dopamine. Most of the environmental factors that inhibit MAO-A, boost MAO-B activity such as stress, lipid peroxidation, high estrogen levels, mercury, aluminum, cadmium, high copper, high levels of hydroxyl ions (9, 32, 33, 34, 35, 36, 37, 38, 39, 40, 41, 42, 43, 44). The accumulative presence of these environmental factors can result in a very low MAO-A:MAO-B ratio and very high MAO-B activity may inhibit the production of cholesterol.

The newer formulation of Respen-A™ known as Respen-A™ Blended Chord has a 4X homeopathic dilution of reserpine and a 12C dilution of a reserpine metabolite. The

Respen-A™ Blended Chord appears to increase MAO-A activity and decrease MAO-B activity. Limited preliminary reports have indicated an increase in total cholesterol levels in a patient with high functioning autism using Respen-A™ Blended Chord. This patient's total cholesterol levels had steadily declined to 95 mg/dL over a 3 year period prior to starting Respen-A™ Blended Chord. Six weeks after starting Respen-A™ Blended Chord the total cholesterol had increased to 113 mg/dL. After 12 weeks on Respen-A™ Blended Chord his total cholesterol increased to 127 mg/dL.

NOTE: Respen-A is a prescription item available from a number of pharmacies in the United States and Canada. To learn more about Respen-A please visit their informative website at www.Respen-A.com.

References:

1. Cohen IL, Liu X, Schutz C, White BN, Jenkins EC, Brown WT, & Holden JJ. (2003, Sept). Association of autism severity with a monoamine oxidase A functional polymorphism. Clin Genet 64(3), pp. 190-197.

2. Davis LK, Hazlett HC, Librant AL, Nopoulos P, Sheffield VC, Piven J, & Wassink TH. (2008, Oct 5). Cortical enlargement in autism is associated with a functional VNTR in the monoamine oxidase A gene. Am J Med Genet B Neuropsychiatr Genet 1478(7), pp. 1145-1151.

3. Contini V, Marques FZ, Garcia CE, Hutz MH, & Bau CH. (2006, Apr 5). MAOA-uVNTR polymorphism in a Brazilian sample: further support for the association with .impulsive behaviors and alcohol dependence. Am J Med Genet B Neuropsychiatry Genet 141B(3), pp. 305-308.

4. Craig IW. (2005). The role of monoamine oxidase A, MAOA, in the aetiology of antisocial behaviour: the importance of gene-environment interactions. Novartis Found Symp 268, pp. 227-237.

5. Alia-Klein N., Goldstein RZ., Kriplani A., Logan J., Tomasi D., Williams B., Telang F., Shumay E., Biegon A., Craig IW., Henn F., Wang GJ., Volkow ND, & Fowler JS. (2008, May 7). Brain Monoamine Oxidase-A Activity Predicts Trait Aggression: Brain MAO-A predicts aggression. J. Neuroscience 28(9), pp. 5099-5104.

6. Youdim M.B.H. & Sandler M. (1968). Activation of monoamine oxidase and inhibition of aldehyde dehyrogenase by reserpine. European Journal of Pharmacology, 4, pp. 105 –108.

7. Vijayalakshmi V, Lele JV, & Daginawala HF. (1978). Effect of reserpine on the monoamine oxidase (MAO) activity in rat liver and brain. Biochemical Pharmacology 27(15), pp. 1985-1986.

8. Lehman E., Haber J., & Lesser S. (1957, July-September). The Use of Reserpine in Autistic Children. The Journal of Nervous and Mental Disease, 125(3), pp. 351-356.

9. Chauhan A, Gu F, Essa M.M., Wegiel J, Kaur K, Brown W.T., & Chauhan V. (2011). Brain region- specific deficit in mitochondrial electron transport chain complexes in children with autism. Neurochem 117(2), pp. 209-220.

10. Launay JM, Ferrari P, Haimart M, Bursztejn C, Tabuteau F, Braconnier A, Pasques-Bondoux D, Luong C, & Dreux C. (1988). Serotonin metabolism and other biochemical parameters in infantile autism. A controlled study of 22 autistic children. Neuropsychobiology 20(1), pp. 1-11.

11. Lake CR, Ziegler MG, & Murphy DL. (1977, May). Increased norepinephrine levels and decreased dopamine-beta-hydroxylase activity in primary autism. Arch Gen Psychiatry 34(5), pp. 553-556.

12. McNamara IM, Borelia AW, Bialowas LA, & Whitaker-Azmitia PM. (2008, Jan 16). Further studies in the developmental hyperserotonemia model (DHS) of autism: social, behavioral and peptide changes. Brain Res 1189, pp. 203-214.

13. Chevillard C, Barden N, & Saavedra J.M. (1981, Oct 5). Estradiol treatment decreases type A and increases type B monoamine oxidase in specific brain stem areas and cerebellum of ovariectomized rats. Brain Research 222(1), pp. 177-181.

14. Jergensen HS. (2007, Nov). Studies on the neuroendocrine role of serotonin. Dan Med Bull 54(4), pp. 266-288.

15. Larsson L.G., Renyi L., Ross S.B., Svensson B., Angeby-Moller K. (1990, Feb). Different effects on the responses of functional pre- and postsynaptic 5-HT1A receptors by repeated treatment of rats with the 5-HT1A receptor agonist 8-OH-DPAT. Neuropharmacology, 29(2), pp. 86-91.

16. Baumann P.A. & Waldmeier P.C., (1984, January). Negative feedback control of serotonin release in vivo: comparison of 5-hydroxyindolacetic acid levels measured by voltammetry in conscious rats and by biochemical techniques. Neuroscience, 11(1), pp. 195-204.

17. Ma Z, Zhang G, Jenney C, Krishnamoorthy S, & Tao R. (2008, July 7). Characterization of serotonin-toxicity syndrome (toxidrome) elicited by 5-hydroxy-l-trytophan in clorgyline-pretreated rats. Eur J Pharmacology 588(2-3), pp. 198-206.

18. Curin JM, Terzic` IM, Petkovic` ZB, Zekan L, Terzic` IM, & Susnjara IM. (2003, August). Lower cortisol and higher ACTH levels in individuals with autism. J Autism Dev Disord 33(4), pp. 443-448.

19. Jabbi, M., Korf, J., Kema, I.P., Hartman, C., van der Pompe, G., Minderaa, R.B., Ormel, J., & den Boer, J.A. (2007, May). Convergent genetic modulation of the endocrine stress response involves polymorphic variations of 5-HTT, COMT and MAOA. Mol Psychiatry, 12(5), pp. 483-490.

20. Marinovic`-Curin J, Marinovic`-Terzic` I, Bujas-Petkovic` Z, Zekan L, Skrabic` V, Dogas Z, & Terzic` J. ((2008, Feb). Slower cortisol response during ACTH stimulation test in autistic children. Eur Child Adolesc Psychiatry 17(1), pp. 39-43.

21. Popova NK, Masiova LN, Morosova EA, Bulygina VV, & Seif I. (2006, Feb). MAO-A knockout attenuates adrenocortical response to various kinds of stress. Psychoneuroendocrinology 31(2), pp. 179-186.

22. Brummett BH, Boyle SH, Siegler IC, Kuhn CM, Surwit RS, Garrett ME, Collins A, Ashley-Koch A, & Williams RB. (2008, Oct). HPA axis function in male caregivers: effect of the monoamine oxidase-A gene promoter (MAOA-uVNTR). Biol Psychol 79(2), pp. 250-255.

23. Hoshino Y, Yokoyama F, Watanabe M, Murata S, Kaneko M, Y Kumashiro H. (1987, June). The diurnal variation and response to dexamethasone suppression test of saliva cortisol level in autistic children. Jpn J Psychiatry Neurol 41(2), pp. 227-235.

24. Jergensen H, Knigge U, Kjaer A, Moller M, & Warberg J. (2002, Oct). Serotonergic stimulation of corticotropin-releasing hormone and proopiomelanocortin gene expression. J Neuroendocrinology 14(10), pp. 788-795.

25. Sandman CA, Touchette P, Marion S, Lenjavi M, & Chicz-Demet A. (2002, Oct 15). Disregulation of proopiomelanocortin and contagious maladaptive behavior. Regul Pept 108(2-3), pp. 179-185.

26. Heron P, Cousins K, Boyd C, & Daya S. (2001, Feb 23). Paradoxical effects of copper and manganese on brain mitochondrial function. Life-Sci 68(14), pp. 1575-1583.

27. Cakala M, Drabik J, Kaz`mierczak A, Kopczuk D, & Adamczyk A. (2006). Inhibition of mitochondrial complex II affects dopamine metabolism and decreases its uptake into striatal synaptosomes. Folia Neuropathol 44(4), pp. 238-243.

28. Gillberg C & Svennerholm L. (1987, July). CSF monoamines in autistic syndromes and other

pervasive developmental disorders of early childhood. Br J Psychiatry 151, pp. 89-94.

29. Dziobek I, Gold SM, Wolf OT, & Convit A. (2007, Jan 15). Hypercholesteremia in Asperger syndrome: independence from lifestyle, obsessive-compulsive behavior, and social anxiety. Psychiatry Res 149(1-3), pp. 321-324.

30. Brummett BH, Boyle SH, Siegler IC, Zuchner S, Ashley-Koch A, & Williams RB. (2008, Feb). Lipid levels are associated with a regulatory polymorphism of the monoamine oxidase-A gene promoter (MAOA-uVNTR). Med Sci Monit 14(2), pp. 57-61.

31. Great Plains Laboratory www.greatplainslaboratory.com/home/eng/full_oat.asp

32. Ma, ZQ., Violani, E., Villa, F., Picotti, GB., & Maggi, A. (1995, September). Estrogenic control of monoamine oxidase A activity in human neuroblastoma cells expressing physiological concentrations of estrogen receptor. European Journal of Pharmacology, 284 (1-2), pp. 171-176.

33. Medvedev A.E., Rajgorodskaya D.I., Gorkin V.Z., Fedotova I.B., & Semiokhina A.F. (1992, February-April). The role of lipid peroxidation in the possible involvement of membrane-bound monoamine oxidases

in gamma-aminobutyric acid and glucosamine deamination in rat brain. Focus on chemical pathogenesis of experimental audiogenic epilepsy. Molecular Chemistry Neuropathology 16(1-2), pp. 187-201.

34. Rao K.S., & Rao G.V. (1994, August, 17). Effect of aluminum (Al) on brain mitochondrial monoamine oxidase-A (MAO-A) activity – an in vitro kinetic study. Molecular and Cellular Biochemistry 137(1), pp. 57-60.

35. Zatta P., Zambenedetti P., & Milanese M. (1999, November, 26). Activation of monoamine oxidase type-B by aluminum in rat brain homogenate. Neuroreport 10(17), pp. 3645-3648.

36. Leung T.K., Lim L., & Lai J.C. (1992, September). Differential effects of metal ions on type A and type B monoamine oxidase activities in rat brain and liver mitochondria. Metabolic Brain Disorders 7(3), pp. 139-146.

37. Narang R.I., Gupta K.R., Narang A.P., & Singh R. (1991, October). Levels of copper and zinc in depression. Indian Journal of Physiology and Pharmacology 35(4), pp. 272-274.

38. Soto-Otero R., Mendez-Alvarez E., Hermida-Ameijeiras A., Sanchez-Sellero I., Cruz-Landeira A.,

& Lamas M.L. (2001, July 13). Inhibition of brain monoamine oxidase activity by the generation of hydroxyl radicals: potential implications in relaxation to oxidative stress. Life Sciences 69(8), pp. 879-889.

39. Clow, A., Patel, S., Najafi, M., Evans, P.D., & Hucklebridge, F. (1997), The cortisol response to psychological challenge is preceded by a transient rise in endogenous inhibitor of monoamine oxidase. Life Science, 61(5), pp. 567-575.

40. Shemyakov, SE., (2001, June). Monoamine oxidase activity, lipid peroxidation, and morphological changes in human hypothalamus during aging. Bulletin of Experimental Biology and Medicine, 131 (6), pp. 586-588.

41. Volchegorskii, IA., Tseilikman, VE., Smirnov, DS., Ship, SA., & Borisenkov, AV. (2004, September). Decreases in glucocorticoid sensitivity as a factor of stress-producing changes in the activity of monoamine oxidase, lipid peroxidation, and behavior in rats. Neurosciense Behavior Physiology, 34 (7), pp. 697-701.

42. Hucklebridge F., Sen S., Evans P.D., & Clow A. (1998). The relationship between circadian patterns of salivary cortisol and endogenous inhibitor of monoamine oxidase A. Life Sciences 62(25), pp. 2321-2328.

43. Doyle A., Hucklebridge F., Evans P., & Clow A. (1996). Salivary monoamine oxidase A and B inhibitory activities correlate with stress. Life Sciences 59(16), pp. 1357-1362.

44. Avgustinovich D.F., Alekseendo O.V., Bakshtanovskaia I.V., Koriakina L.A., Lipina T.V., Tenditnik M.V., Bondar' N.P., Kovalenko I.L., & Kudriavtseva N.N. (2004, October-December). Dynamic changes of brain serotonergic and dopaminergic activities during development of anxious depression: experimental study. Usp Fiziol Nauk 35(4), pp. 19-40.

Additional Information

Getting Children To Take Supplements

By Lori Knowles (New Beginnings Nutritionals)

Starting nutritional supplement therapy with children can be very stressful for parents. Children with developmental disabilities (such as ADD/HD, Autism, Sensory Integration Dysfunction, etc.) may be required by physicians to take anywhere from 6 to 20 different nutritional supplements each day. This can be overwhelming to parents, especially when their children do not swallow pills and strongly resist being forced to consume anything that is not of their choosing.

Many parents ask me about products in chewable or liquid form. Although there are a few good liquid and/or chewable supplement products available that are appropriate for kids with autism/special needs, they can be expensive and children can still object to the taste.

Below are some suggestions that have been tried by parents to help overcome the problem of their children running away, clenching their teeth, and spitting back out what is put into their mouths. Whether the supplements you are giving are in capsule, liquid, or chewable form, following these six steps should help with getting your child to comply.

1. **Take a No-Nonsense Approach.** Give supplements with the same level of intensity that you use to give them a life-saving medication. Your child needs these supplements to support their brain, immune system and overall nutritional status. Your child can sense when you mean business and you cannot allow them to think that taking their supplements are optional.

2. **Do not mix into food or drink and pretend that it's not there!** This only works if you are adding only one or two tasteless supplements. Even if they can't taste it they may choose not to finish the drink or food that it's mixed in and the child is not getting everything they need. As you add more needed supplements to their regimen, hiding them in food will eventually backfire. The last thing we want children who are picky eaters to do is to stop eating because they are suspicious of what may have been added to their food.

3. **Choose the Best Method for your Child to Administer Supplements.** You need to take into effect the sensory/swallowing issues that your child has. Does your child do better with liquids or semi-solids? The two most common mediums in which to mix supplements are fruit purees or liquids.

    Fruit purees/baby food: I chose baby food as a way to get supplements into my child because he loved the fruit purees as a baby – especially the peaches. The tartness of the peaches is especially good because it masks the taste of a lot of supplements – especially the B vitamins. I sometimes rotated with pears and applesauce as well. I would recommend using organic baby food or making your own because of pesticide residues in these foods. Open up each capsule and mix in into the fruit puree of choice (1-2 tbsp). Add one drop of stevia to sweeten and additionally mask the supplement taste, if needed.

Liquids: For children who have a problem with the taste and texture of fruit purees, use a tart or strong juice and pour a small amount (1-2 tbsp) into a bowl. Open up and empty supplement capsules into the bowl and mix well with your finger to dissolve as much as possible. While the mixture is still swirling, use a large syringe to suck up the supplement mixture. If possible, use only enough liquid to fill one syringe, two at most.

Some examples of juices/liquids that parents are using to mix supplements in include: pear, pineapple, orange, grape, Sunny Delight, water, or a small amount of favorite soda. It is recommended that you only use 1-2 tablespoons of liquid and only use the liquids of choice for giving supplements, not for regular drinks in order to avoid confusion.

Remember that the choice of liquids or purees used should be based upon *your* child's issues which need to take into consideration any allergies, phenol sensitivities, and sensitivity to sugar. **Adding one drop of liquid stevia (Wisdom Natural brand**

166

recommended) can add additional sweetness (without feeding yeast) to further mask the taste of supplements.

4. <u>Use the Concept of "First – Then."</u> This is a critical concept to ensure compliance. If your child is in an ABA program, this would be a good place to learn this concept. Otherwise, parents can reinforce this concept by repeating it in everyday life experiences (i.e. first we turn on the water, than we wash our hands). Even a very young child can learn this concept if it's repeated enough. Once this concept is understood, you need to consistently use it enforce compliance. Next, choose a favorite activity (eating the next meal, watching video/TV, favorite toy, blanket, etc), for the purpose of withholding it until or AFTER the child takes the supplements successfully. For example: "Daniel, do you want to <u>(eat breakfast)</u>? FIRST you must take your (vitamins, medicines, or any name you want to call it that you use every time) BEFORE you can <u>(eat breakfast)</u>. Even today, if my son decides to delay or give me trouble with taking his supplements, I turn off the TV and tell him that it stays off until the supplements are swallowed.
It is important to **be firm and never waiver** on this, because it will ensure that success will come quickly.

5. <u>Use Rewards to Associate Good with the Bad.</u> This comes in handy when a child needs extra reinforcement. Another useful approach to further ensure compliance is to give a reward, which only comes immediately after the child successfully taking the supplements. ALWAYS give lots of praise and hugs as well as one good tasting reward that they can

associate with taking yucky supplements. I have used good tasting chewable vitamin C tablets (only buffered C recommended) because more vitamin C is always good for the child, and it may taste somewhat like "candy" to them. Other options could include Juice Plus gummies, a small piece of Health Food Store (HFS) fruit leather or gummy bear, or even a very small drink of a favorite soda. Remember that it is important to not go overboard and load your child up with sugar (fruit sugar included), which can aggravate or cause yeast overgrowth.

6. **Be consistent and firm.** If you are firm and do not give in to the conditions you set down for your child, most children will start to comply within 2-3 days because they know that they cannot win the battle. Wait them out for as long as you need to, and when they FINALLY give in and take the supplements, quickly give them praise, the preferred activity and the small reward that is given every time they successfully take their supplements. This positive reinforcement will encourage them to be more willing next time.

How To Successfully Work With a Biomedical Autism Doctor

These suggestions have been acquired over the years in my practice and have helped me assist my patients. Also, in talking with many other doctors working with families of a loved one with autism these recommendations often hold true as well.

- Journal – keep a running journal of your observations and timeline of therapies you are implementing.
- Keep a spreadsheet of therapies.
- Keep dates of when new therapies such as when supplements were started, stopped, and what reactions were seen (good or bad).
- Recognize your child's patterns – situational, seasonal, time of day.
- If added new therapies and problems are seen – then cut out some or all new therapies giving before reactions occurred, then reintroduce slowly to isolate which one was the potential culprit. Notify your doctor of these changes.
- You will need to become a detective of your child's particular autism condition.
- You know your child better than anyone – be involved 100%.
- You are ultimately responsible for your own health and your child's health care.

- Be prepared for your consultations with questions, concerns, and important topics you want to cover. Have these sent via fax or email prior to your consult.
- Ask whether your practitioner receives faxes, emails, or voice mail regarding questions. Be prepared to pay for extra time. Most doctors will answer questions that are related to a new therapy introduced or quick follow-up questions to a recent visit
- Partnering with your practitioner also means having a relationship with the office staff. Treat them with respect. They are there to help.
- Do not assume your doctor remembers every detail about your child – *keep them informed.*
- If you change supplements by either removing or adding them let your practitioner know in writing via fax or email. This way they can keep a copy for their records.
- Come prepared with your latest observations about your child.
- Let your doctor know what different therapies, testing, etc. you want to explore.
- Keep a running list of supplements, medications, calendar of therapy implementation, reactions to therapies.
- Let your doctor know when you have sent off tests or if you are having problems getting tests samples collected. Some offices track follow-up appointments based on incoming tests.

Critical Point: The parents and/or care-givers who are most successful in implementing biomedical therapies for their children are the ones who are 100% committed to the process.

Some Thoughts on Heavy Metal Toxicity

Heavy metal toxicity is a serious issue and needs to be approached comprehensively. There is a tremendous amount of confusion about what heavy metal toxicity means for an autism-spectrum child, and the best ways of approaching the removal of these toxins. The one word that causes a lot of confusion is "chelation" which means "to bind" in Latin. It is a chemical term that describes a particular chemical bond that occurs when a metal or other mineral is surrounded or attached to a binding agent.

Unfortunately, the word conjures up images of metal and minerals being aggressively ripped from cells leaving behind shredded fragments of cellular debris. To others it sounds similar to chemotherapy and the fears of toxicity are created. Because of this I (and other doctors) like to use heavy metal detoxification (HMD) to better describe the process of heavy metal removal. Just remember that when you hear the word chelation it is in reference to the process of removing heavy metals with particular medications.

There is also a lot of confusion (and fear) surrounding the issue of HMD in general. Many in the traditional medical community think that it is unwarranted to treat children with autism with HMD – stating that there is no proof it is effective or useful. Also, mainstream medicines notion that HMD is extremely toxic to autism-spectrum children creates

171

a lot of conflicting ideas about the benefits of HMD. This section is not meant to be an in-depth discussion about HMD and all the various protocols that exist for doing this. What I want to point out is the following:

- Heavy metal detoxification is the medically approved therapy for heavy metal poisoning – mercury, lead.
- HMD has been used all over the world for heavy metal toxicity.
- There is no other treatment for heavy metal toxicity than HMD – it is the treatment of choice, other than do nothing.
- Heavy metal toxicity is real – it is a proven medical condition.
- Any drug has the potential for toxicity.
- Any patient has the potential for allergic reactions.
-

Ask yourself one question:
"Is the presence of heavy metals in your child's body safe?"

Heavy Metal Detoxification is NOT a specific treatment for autism

- HMD is a treatment for heavy metal poisoning – regardless of a person's diagnosis.
- ASD children are likely to benefit because they are neurologically impaired, and heavy metals such as mercury and lead are often found to be elevated.

What is the medically approved treatment for heavy metal poisoning/toxicity for people with the following conditions?

- Alzheimer's Disease
- Asthma
- Brain Cancer
- Chronic Fatigue
- Diabetes
- Gout
- High Blood Pressure
- Lupus
- Multiple Sclerosis

You guessed it – HMD. If a doctor finds that a patient with cancer is lead poisoned what do you think should happen? That patient should be treated for the lead toxicity. If that patient with cancer got strep throat do you think a doctor is not going to treat it? Of course not!

Why HMD Is Not More Recognized - Why Is It So Controversial?

- Most doctors are taught very little about heavy metal toxicity in medical school other than lead toxicity.
- Most doctors do not know what to look for regarding heavy metal toxicity, and even more know nothing about the various treatment protocols.

Most medical authorities live in a small box – heavy metal toxicity is not high on the list for things to learn about.

The Bottom Line Regarding HMD

- Any doctor or person who tells you HMD is dangerous, toxic and should be avoided for ASD children knows nothing about the biomedical underpinnings of autism.
- They also likely know nothing about toxicity factors.
- More than likely they have never implemented heavy metal treatment for a patient and are speaking out of ignorance.
- HMD is the treatment of choice for heavy metal toxicity – just as:
    - Antibiotics are the treatment of choice for Strep Throat, or
    - Insulin injections are for insulin-dependent diabetics.
    - …etc.

No one can convince you that the biomedical approach, including heavy metal detoxification therapy for your autism-spectrum child is worthwhile. You must come to this conclusion yourself. Become empowered and educate yourself. Make informed decisions regarding your child's care!

How Quickly Will Some Therapies Start Working?

Everyone wants to see positive changes happen with their children when they implement biomedical therapy. Having some level of expectation and appreciation for average time frames give a parent or care giver a reference point for what to expect. Of course, these are only estimates, and each child is different, so even if positive changes are not seen early on it doesn't specifically mean benefits will not be achieved over time.

Immediate Feedback Therapies

With many individual's positive changes (improved attention, better eye contact, more social, etc.) can be seen quite rapidly - within 2 to 6 Weeks, on average 4 weeks:

- Medical diets (GF/CF, anti-yeast, phenol reduced)
- Basic nutritional supplements – multi-vitamins and minerals, B-vitamins, essential fatty acids, calcium/magnesium.
- Methylation support – Methyl-B12, DMG, Folinic Acid
- Treating yeast (and bacteria)
- Respen-A

Long-term Feedback

With many individual's positive changes are seen within 6 to 8 weeks, sometimes 2 to 6 months…or more.

- Heavy metal detoxification
- Anti-viral therapy – Valtrex, natural antivirals
- Traditional Hyperbaric Oxygen Therapy (HBOT) – clinic based which is normally done over a few month period of time.

IMPORTANT: These are meant to be viewed as generalizations and NOT absolutes. Every child and their treatment response are different. Just because a therapy is listed as immediate feedback does not mean it will not give long-term benefits, and vice versa. In some cases antiviral or heavy metal detoxification and HBOT can give immediate, recognizable benefits.

Important Points to Always Remember

- You will need to become a detective of your child's particular autism condition.
- You know your child better than anyone – be involved 100%.
- You are ultimately responsible for your own health and your child's health care.
- Stop listening to "nay-sayers and skeptics" no matter who they are like family, friends, or medical professionals. Skeptics create fear, doubt and confusion, and likely know no nothing about the benefits of biomedical treatments for autism.
- Follow your instincts and intuition.
- Be open-minded and hopeful. There is definitely a lot of room for hope for you, your child and your family through biomedical intervention for autism.
- Be patient, persistent and dedicated to the pursuit of wellness for your child.
- Educate yourself in the field of biomedical intervention for autism.

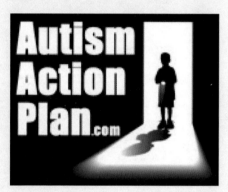

Autism Supplements

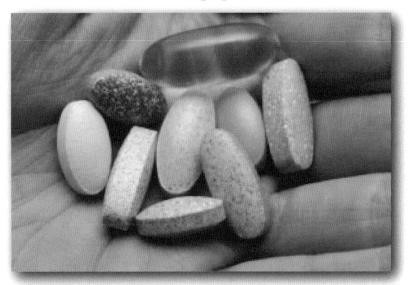

Supplements are an important element in treating the various issues many individuals on the autism–spectrum have, including nutritional deficiencies, speech and language disorder, mood instability, sensory issues, focusing and attention problems and others.

- Supplements Designed Specifically For Autism Intervention

- Informative Videos Explaining The Benefits of Specific Supplements.

- Cross Referenced by Supplement Name & What They Help Treat.

www.AutismSupplementsCenter.com

Autism Supplements Guide Book

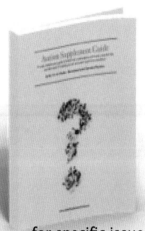

Dr. Woeller's Autism Supplements Guide book is unique in that it not only allows you to learn about individual supplements helpful for autism, but also provides the ability to cross–reference useful supplements for specific issues. It's like having two reference books in one! The content in this 86 page guide book is not a bunch of "theory," or "perfect world" scenarios. Dr. Woeller specifically wrote this to be a user–friendly, "real world" manual that helps guide you through the often complicated and confusing world of supplements and vitamins, and how they relate to autism treatment.

This unique book will also give you supplement dosing recommendations based on Dr. Woeller's 12+ years experience as a clinical as well as biomedical autism physician.

- *What Supplements Should You Use?*
- *What Are The Dosing Recommendations For Various Supplements?*
- *When Do You Give Them?*
- *Is It Important To Combine Supplements?*
- *What Supplements Shouldn't Be Taken With Others?*
- *What Benefits Can You Expect To See From Autism Supplements?*
- *What Side Effects Might There Be?*

Get It Now!
www.AutismSupplementsCenter.com/Guide-Book/

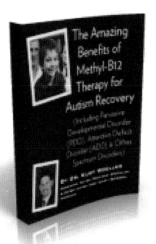

Autism Video Lab Reviews

Don't Understand These?

Get A Video Test Results
Review & Interpretation by
Dr. Kurt Woeller!

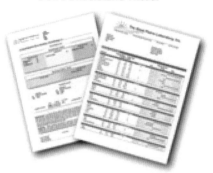

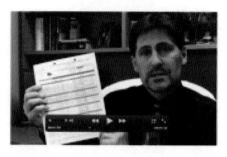

"What Do All Those Lines And Graphs Mean On My Test Results?"

 It can be very confusing trying to decipher all the test markers by yourself, and then what are you supposed to with the information?

We can help. Send your test results to us, and our doctor will analyze and review the test results, record it, and send you the link to the video.

www.AutismVideoLabReviews.com

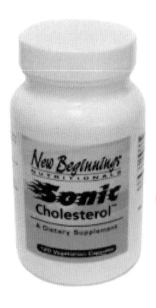

Cholesterol Test Reviews & Sonic Cholesterol Supplementation

Did You Know Low Cholesterol Levels Can Be Just as Dangerous as High Cholesterol Levels?

We have been told for years that cholesterol levels being too high are problematic, that it can contribute to heart disease and strokes. In fact, this is true for many people. However, what has gone unrecognized or ignored for many years is that too low cholesterol can be just as detrimental, often leading to a myriad of mental health and disease conditions. There is a dynamic balance of all things in the body that must be achieved for optimal health to manifest, and cholesterol is a critically important component of that balance.

Sonic Cholesterol is an excellent choice for reviving low cholesterol levels. Sonic Cholesterol is a pure and potent nutritional supplement designed specifically to support healthy cholesterol levels. Sonic Cholesterol is the only cholesterol supplement on the market designed to help raise cholesterol to normal levels.

www.GetSonicCholesterol.com

Index

About the Author

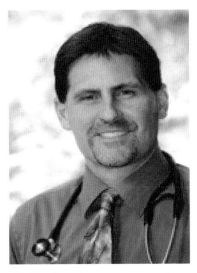

Kurt N. Woeller, D.O., has been a complementary medicine physician and biomedical autism specialist since 1998. He is an author, lecturer, clinical practitioner and medical director for **Sunrise Complementary Medical Center** offering specialized treatment and testing for individuals with complex medical conditions like autism, Chronic Fatigue Syndrome and Fibromyalgia, mental health disorders, Multiple Sclerosis, and other chronic health disorders. Dr. Woeller serves as a clinical consultant for both **BioHealth** and **Great Plains Laboratory** providing patient and physician education through training programs and monthly webinars. Dr. Woeller has lectured nationwide regarding the benefits of biomedical therapies for chronic health disorders. He currently runs an extensive educational resource for parents of autistic children at www.AutismActionPlan.com. You can also visit his main resource website at www.DrWoeller.com.

Made in the USA
San Bernardino, CA
05 July 2014